PRAISE FOR
# *WHAT YOUR DOCTOR MAY NOT TELL YOU ABOUT*™ *DEPRESSION*

"The definitive work on integrative approaches to depression from one of the true deans of complementary medicine. I've been practicing for over twenty years, and I still look to Dr. Schachter as one of my mentors."

—Ronald Hoffman, MD, author of
*How to Talk to Your Physician*, and host of
*Health Talk* on the WOR Radio Network

"This book's practical and effective nutritional strategies—from a leader in the holistic health field—offer a lifeline to all those caught in our epidemic of depression."

—Julia Ross, MA, executive director,
Recovery Systems Clinic, and
author of *The Mood Cure*

"In this book, Schachter and Mitchell challenge us to imagine the problem of depression differently. They make a strong scientific case for their view. I hope this book will be read as widely as it truly deserves, by clinicians as well as sufferers of depression."

—Majid Ali, MD, author of
*The Principles and Practice of Integrative Medicine*

*Please turn the page for more reviews . . .*

"An excellent overview of the multiple causes of depression and the many opportunities for effective treatment."
—Richard A. Kunin, MD, president,
Society for Orthomolecular Health Medicine; and
diplomate, American Board of Psychiatry and Neurology

"Dr. Schachter astutely points out many factors that may contribute to depression and provides a comprehensive integrative approach . . . The health of those suffering from depression will almost certainly benefit from the application of the knowledge contained in this book."
—Kenneth A. Bock, MD, author of *Road to Immunity*,
cofounder and codirector, Rhinebeck Health Center,
Rhinebeck, New York

"This book fills a very important need . . . I can't imagine how any physician can practice proper diagnosis and treatment of mood disorders without knowing what is in this book. It is a must for all practitioners and healers."
—A. Hoffer, MD, PhD, FRCP(C)

"Dr. Schachter not only stresses the very significant problems with psychotropic drugs, but also provides a number of safe, highly effective alternatives for the treatment of depression."
—Julian Whitaker, MD, author of
*Health & Healing* newsletter and founder,
The Whitaker Wellness Institute

# WHAT YOUR DOCTOR MAY *NOT* TELL YOU ABOUT™

# DEPRESSION

## The Breakthrough Integrative Approach for Effective Treatment

MICHAEL B. SCHACHTER, MD,
medical director, the Schachter Center for
Complementary Medicine

with DEBORAH MITCHELL

A Lynn Sonberg Book

**WARNER
WELLNESS**

NEW YORK   BOSTON

PUBLISHER'S NOTE: The information herein is not intended to replace the services of trained health professionals or be a substitute for medical advice. You are advised to consult with your health care professional with regard to matters relating to your health, and in particular regarding matters that may require diagnosis or medical attention.

Warner Wellness
Hachette Book Group USA
1271 Avenue of the Americas, New York, NY 10020
Visit our Web site at www.HachetteBookGroupUSA.com.

The title of the series What Your Doctor May *Not* Tell You About . . . and the related trade dress are trademarks owned by Warner Books, Inc., and may not be used without permission.

Warner Wellness is an imprint of Warner Books, Inc.

Warner Wellness is a trademark of Time Warner Inc. or an affiliated company. Used under license by Hachette Book Group USA, which is not affiliated with Time Warner Inc.

Printed in the United States of America

First Edition: November 2006
10   9   8   7   6   5   4   3   2   1

Library of Congress Cataloging-in-Publication Data
Schachter, Michael B.
    What your doctor may not tell you about depression / Michael B. Schachter, and Deborah Mitchell.— 1st ed.
       p. cm.
    Includes index.
    ISBN-13: 978-0-446-69494-0
    ISBN-10: 0-446-69494-0
  1. Depression, Mental—Popular works. 2. Depression, Mental—Alternative treatment.
I. Mitchell, Deborah R. II. Title.
    RC537.S378 2006
    616.85'27—dc22                         2005035373

*Cover design by Diane Luger*
*Book design by Charles A. Sutherland*

This book is dedicated to my wife, Lisa, who during the past thirteen years has offered me support and nurturance, and to all of my children: Brian and his wife, Lisa, and their son and my grandson, Eidan; Amy (who was the inspiration for the path that I took in my medical career); Stefan and his fiancée, Alisha; Adam; Jason; and Seth. All of them have played a role in my understanding of people and how to help them.

# Acknowledgments

————— ❦ —————

I'd like to acknowledge and thank Deborah Mitchell for her tireless efforts in helping me to express my ideas and put them into a readable form. She exhibited a real talent for simplifying and integrating the material that we present.

My patients are a constant source of inspiration and knowledge. With the development of the Internet, they continue to alert me to new things on the horizon and help me to refine and improve my approach to helping people.

I thank my colleagues and staff at the Schachter Center for their devotion and stimulation, challenging me to constantly improve our diagnostic and treatment procedures. I especially would like to thank my physician assistants, Sally Minniefield (who has been with me for more than thirty years) and John Reynolds (who has been with me for twenty-five years); my head nurse, Dolores Tritico (who has been with me for twenty-five years); acupuncturist Bob Connolly (who has been at the Schachter Center for eighteen years and helped with the energy section of the book); Peter Reznik, whose approach to managing stress with his unique imaging techniques helped with certain portions of the book; and Sandra Davis (who has managed the store at the Center for many years, is a Reiki master, and helped with the energy section of the book on Reiki).

Our nutrition counselors, Lee Clifford and Anita Berger, helped patients to improve their diets and were always there for questions to help me clarify my thinking. Our office manager, Gabrielle Clenin, and assistant office managers Deborah

McGovern and Jeri Castelluccio have always been there for support and fresh ideas.

My wife, Lisa (a nurse and nurse practitioner), who has worked for years at the Center as a nurse and who has offered constant behind-the-scenes support to our staff, and continues to help out, though she now teaches nursing full-time at a local community college. She also has helped me to be less verbose and to simplify.

I also want to thank other staff members at the Schachter Center who continue to help the Center function well and most of all show caring and concern for all of our patients. Sue Anello, who has consulted at the Schachter Center, is a classically trained homeopath who helped with the energy section of the book.

Friends and family have also been a great source of support. I'd like to thank my sons Jason and Seth Schachter for reading portions of the book and offering me some feedback. Marlene Schachter (a psychiatric social worker) also read portions of the book and offered some good suggestions. Peggy Muller always had good questions about how things work and stimulated my thinking, especially about the role of Lyme disease in some patients with mood disorders.

My colleagues and friends in orthomolecular psychiatry and complementary, alternative and integrative medicine have been a constant inspiration and resource to help clarify my ideas about helping patients. I want to thank the organization American College for Advancement in Medicine (ACAM) for being a leader in the new approach to health care and the source and/or inspiration for much of my knowledge during the past thirty years.

Finally, I am indebted to Lynn Sonberg, who asked me to write this book and helped to keep me in line in terms of deadlines and helped me write a book for the public.

# Contents

# Introduction

---------------- ❦ ----------------

As I sit down to write this book, the Food and Drug Administration (FDA) has just approved another antidepressant. The name of the drug doesn't matter; it joins the ranks of about one dozen others already on the market. Presently, more than two dozen additional antidepressants are under development, according to the trade group Pharmaceutical Research and Manufacturers of America. And as you sit today and read this book, another antidepressant has been, is being, or soon will be released to the market, to be followed by others currently in research-and-development or trial phases.

While the good intentions of those who work so diligently to find remedies for the millions of people who suffer with depression may be commendable, I remain largely unimpressed. Why? Because regardless of the number of antidepressants introduced to the market or when they appear, the bottom line is that *psychotropic drugs are not the complete answer to the critical and growing problem of depression in this country. In fact, I believe that in some ways they contribute to it.*

On the surface, these statements may seem daunting and depressing. After all, we've been told by the conventional medical community, the pharmaceutical companies, and Madison

Avenue marketers that drugs will lift your spirits, improve your mood, and spark up your sex life.

If drugs are not the answer, then what is? There is no simple answer to this question, but there *is* an approach to helping people with depression that has largely been ignored by conventional psychiatry. I and a growing number of my colleagues have found it to be a natural, biofriendly approach called orthomolecular psychiatry—the practice of treating psychological problems by providing the body with optimal amounts of substances that are natural to it—including amino acids, vitamins and minerals, trace elements, and essential fatty acids—combined with positive lifestyle habits and mind–body therapies. Linus Pauling, PhD, originally introduced this term in 1968 in the journal *Science*.

In this book I explain how you or a loved one, and the tens of millions of Americans who suffer with depression and related disorders, can find relief naturally, safely, and effectively, without the use of medication. This approach has worked for tens of thousands of individuals, and it can work for you, too. I see proof of it every day at my center, the Schachter Center for Complementary Medicine in Suffern, New York. You don't need to come to Suffern to win your battle against depression, but you *do* need to take your healing process into your own hands, and that's what I can help you do with this book.

I was introduced to the compelling and dramatic capabilities of orthomolecular medicine in the early 1970s, when I heard of several cases in which individuals who suffered with clotting problems were treated successfully with vitamin E. My interest was piqued, and as I read what little but impressive literature there was on the subject, I also learned that some children with brain damage had been helped with vitamin E therapy. This information hit home, because my two-and-a-half-year-old daughter suffered from cerebral palsy. Despite intensive, daily rehabilitation, she had not progressed past crawling on her belly. I began to give her 100 International Units (IU) of vitamin E daily, and her energy and awareness levels increased within days. After three weeks, I doubled the dose, and within hours she responded by getting up on all fours and rocking back and forth. When I gave vitamin E to her mother, who was pregnant at the time and complaining of fatigue, her energy level improved significantly. I felt I was onto something big.

At the time, I was a conventionally trained, board-certified psychiatrist, and I began to wonder whether a nutritional approach in general—and nutritional supplements in particular—might be able to help my psychiatric patients. The more I explored the world of orthomolecular psychiatry, the more I saw how this approach might hold the answers to many of the medical problems that plague humankind today, including depression and related disorders. Indeed, some of the most convincing work in orthomolecular psychiatry occurred in the 1950s with Abram Hoffer, PhD, who, along with several colleagues, discovered that adding niacin (vitamin $B_3$) in high doses to the treatment of schizophrenic patients significantly improved results. Since then, said Dr. Hoffer in *Vitamin B-3 and Schizophrenia*, "orthomolecular psychiatry has evolved from a simple use of one vitamin for treating one disease to a comprehensive holistic program which includes use of many different nutrients, in combination with standard psychiatric treatment."

Gradually, I became more and more convinced that using only conventional psychiatric medications and psychotherapy was insufficient to treat depression and related disorders. In addition, this approach is fraught with problems because of the adverse side effects of the medications and the failure to address issues relevant to the development of depression and other psychiatric conditions. So how much of a problem is depression in the United States? The following facts are sobering:

- Depression affects more than nineteen million Americans in a given year.
- Ten percent of young people are depressed.
- Major depression is the leading cause of disability in the United States.
- Depression costs an estimated $40 billion each year in lost production, medical costs, and loss of life.
- In 2003, US doctors wrote 213 million prescriptions for antidepressants.
- Many people who are prescribed antidepressants stop taking them because the side effects are too debilitating.
- Two-thirds of people who are depressed never seek or receive treatment, and so suffer needlessly, and about 50 percent of people with chronic depression who do receive treatment do not get sufficient relief. One study (*Journal of the American Medical Association*, June 18, 2003) found an even more disturbing result: Of the people with major depression who sought help, only 22 percent received adequate treatment. (Of course, the adequate treatment referred to in this article consists primarily of antidepressant drugs. As you will see, I agree with the notion that many depressed people are not getting the help they deserve, but this help involves much more than just antidepressant drugs—which in

many cases may not be needed when the other issues discussed in this book are addressed.)

Every one of these points gives us reason to pause, but it may be the last two that are the most distressing. You or someone you love may be part of these staggering statistics; this book can help change that. Here I present effective treatments that are as accessible as changing your diet, supplement habits, and lifestyle, a multifaceted approach designed to bring emotional, mental, physical, and spiritual harmony back into your life often without the use of drugs. This approach is also helpful for related conditions, such as obsessive-compulsive disorder, eating disorders, anxiety disorders, and alcoholism.

## HOW TO USE THIS BOOK

This book is divided into two parts. In part 1, "Coming to Terms with Depression," I talk about what depression is, what causes it, and where to begin to get help. Such a discussion may seem elementary, but it is critical, because many people carry misconceptions about depression, its causes, and how to treat it. For many, the major (or only) way to treat it is to take antidepressant medication. This is understandable since the vast majority of information we've been given about depression has come from those with a vested interest in medication — from pharmaceutical companies to advertising firms and doctors who write prescriptions for these drugs. There is very little discussion about the various alternatives that I will be addressing in this book. Thus, in the first few chapters I try to set the record straight by:

- Comparing the conventional and orthomolecular approaches to treatment of depression and the merits and limits of each.
- Exploring briefly the many causes of and contributors to depression.
- Introducing some tools, including checklists and tests, to help you identify which natural approaches to treatment may work best for you.

Armed with those tools and information, you are now ready to begin work in part 2, "How to Prevent and Treat Depression Comprehensively." In this section, you will learn how different approaches—amino acids, essential fatty acids and other fats, nutrients and herbs, nutritious food, hormones—work to fight depression, and how to use the checklists from chapter 3 to identify which methods are most likely to improve your mood. Because treating depression requires a multifaceted, holistic approach, I also devote several chapters to three other essential areas:

- How to remove dangerous toxins from the body.
- How to fight depression by modifying lifestyle habits.
- How to incorporate energy medicine and personal growth elements into the healing process.

I also devote a chapter to antidepressant and other psychotropic medications, which remain an option, along with the various alternatives discussed in this book. This frank discussion includes their characteristics, benefits, and potential side effects. In this chapter, I also discuss how medications can be added to a natural regimen of amino acids, essential fatty acids, and other natural approaches, if and when necessary. Finally, the book concludes with three success stories, just a few of the many tales from people who have found answers to their depression by using several of the ideas discussed in this book.

Following the text of the book, I have supplied some additional tools. These include:

- Selected notes that supply some references to the text.
- An appendix that lists a variety of resources for further information and further help.
- A glossary in which many terms introduced in the text are defined.
- A suggested reading list for further information on various topics discussed in this book.

As you read this book, I'd like you to keep several points in mind. First, each of us is somewhat different in many ways, including our biochemistry. This notion of biochemical individuality was emphasized by Roger Williams, PhD, in several books back in the 1940s and 1950s. Therefore, it is very important for you to learn to pay attention and listen to your own body. What is good and right for one person may not be good or right for you. Your individual reactions are the key authority, and you must always consider them when evaluating any treatment concepts.

With regard to terminology, I will be using the term *orthomolecular* throughout this book, but some other terms have also been applied to approaches to health care that deviate from conventional medicine. These include *alternative medicine, complementary medicine, alternative and complementary medicine, integrative medicine, functional medicine, environmen-*

*tal medicine, naturopathic medicine,* and *holistic medicine.* Each has a slightly different meaning and different emphasis, but they all have in common that they use a model or approach different from the conventional approach to health care.

Joseph Campbell once said, "If you are following your bliss, you are enjoying that . . . life within you, all the time." Everyone deserves an opportunity to follow their bliss. If you are in the throes of depression, bliss seems unattainable. But when you break free, anything is possible. This book is about possibilities. I encourage you to explore them with me.

*Part   1*

———— ❧ ————

# COMING TO TERMS
# WITH DEPRESSION

# Chapter 1

*⁕*

# What's Wrong with the Mainstream Approach to Treating Depression

If you listen to the pharmaceutical companies and the television and magazine ads, you'd think there's no better time to be depressed in America. Feeling blue? There's a pill just for you. Have you lost interest in your family and friends? Just ask your doctor for the latest tablet. Has your sex drive gone south? Don't worry, there are drugs with a "minimum" of sexual side effects. And if today's new drug or formulation doesn't do the trick, there are dozens more antidepressants in the works.

Treatment of depression has gone the way of treatment of obesity in America: The more diet pills, diet plans, and diet books are made available to the public, the fatter we get. Similarly, as more and more antidepressants are brought to the marketplace, and doctors write more and more prescriptions (more than 213 million in 2003 for antidepressants alone), *the number of people who are depressed continues to climb.* (An in-depth explanation of depression, which is characterized by extreme sadness or low mood and various other specific criteria, is presented in chapter 3.) More than nineteen million Americans are depressed at any one time—and that's a conservative estimate according to some experts, who put the number closer to forty million. Clearly, something is wrong with the way we approach treating depression. In this chapter, I'm going to discuss some elements that have been ignored by mainstream psychiatry and suggest that dealing with them might improve how we handle depression.

One telling example of the magnitude and severity of the problem of depression and related disorders in America can be illustrated by looking at our youth. In a recent study published in the *Archives of Pediatrics and Adolescent Medicine*, researchers stated that prescriptions for children and adolescents with mood and/or behavioral disorders had doubled and in some cases tripled from 1987 through 1996. The use of Prozac-like drugs for children increased 74 percent between 1995 and 1999, according to IMS Health, a global source for pharmaceutical market analysis and information. The use of mood stabilizers in the same population rose 4,000 percent, and prescriptions for newer antipsychotic drugs increased nearly 300 percent.

Perhaps even more revealing examples are the people I see in my practice, people such as Claudia, a thirty-one-year-old receptionist who had been taking antidepressants for years without getting adequate relief. When she came to my center, we uncovered a previously undiagnosed thyroid condition that was contributing to her depression, prescribed low-dose thyroid hormones, developed a nutritional plan for her, and weaned her off her medications. Within weeks she was, in her words, "a completely new person."

There are others like Roger, a forty-four-year-old bank

executive, who came to the center complaining of deep depression, fatigue, insomnia, and loss of sex drive. Roger had been taking various antidepressants and antianxiety drugs on and off for about two years, but the side effects and the lack of appreciable results had discouraged him until he didn't know where to turn. Fortunately, his wife steered him in our direction, and after a thorough evaluation, we treated him with amino acid therapy, essential fatty acids, a vitamin regimen, and acupuncture for stress management and insomnia. Within a month, he was off all his medications and beginning to enjoy life again.

So let's take a look at depression and the brain, so that we can begin to see how the methods used to help these patients worked.

## DEPRESSION AND THE BRAIN

At its core, on a cellular level, *depression is the result of a chemical imbalance in the brain, an imbalance that includes dozens of substances*, each of which plays a role on a continuum that ranges from minor to major, and most of them interacting in some way with the others. This simple definition alone illustrates why treating depression with a single medication or supplement alone is highly unlikely to provide relief.

Among the substances that play a role in causing depression when they are out of balance are chemicals called *neurotransmitters*. Remember this term, because you'll see it a lot in this book.

The living brain is a buzz of activity, where electrical signals pass back and forth among the hundred billion specialized nerve cells, called *neurons*, that make up the brain. Neurons release neurotransmitters for the purpose of transmitting electrical signals, or messages, between neurons. The neurotransmitters leave a neuron and cross a space, called a *synapse*, and attach themselves to various receptor sites on other nearby neurons (see figure below). When a receiving neuron has enough of its receptor sites activated by neurotransmitter molecules, it sends on an electrical signal. This action in turn triggers the transmission of more signals, and the process keeps repeating itself. The firing of multiple brain cells in groups known as *neuronal networks* in a synchronized manner affects what we experience as emotions, thoughts, and sensations.

## Synapse

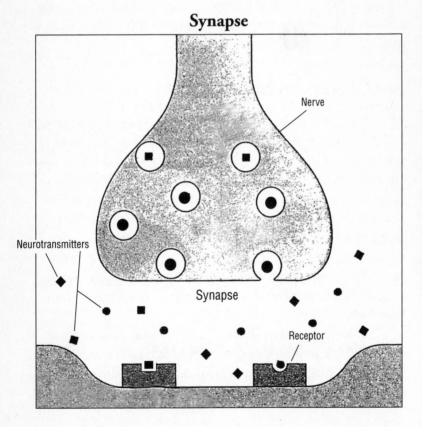

Once neurotransmitter molecules have activated receptor sites, most of them do an about-face, go back across the synapse, and reenter the neuron that originally secreted them. They then may be used to initiate another signal. Later, I will discuss a group of antidepressant drugs whose main action is to block this reentering action (known as *reuptake*), leaving more neurotransmitters in the synapse to carry on their activity. An example of this is the selective serotonin reuptake inhibitors (or SSRIs), whose prototype is Prozac (fluoxetine).

Depression may occur when some neurotransmitters that affect mood are not delivered correctly between neurons, which can happen for a variety of reasons. One reason could be that the levels of one or more neurotransmitters may be too low, making it difficult for neurons to release sufficient amounts of them. In fact, *neurotransmitter deficiency is a very common problem and a major cause of depression.* Another reason may be that the body is unable to reabsorb the neurotransmitters properly or is metabolizing them too thoroughly, leaving them ineffective when the next signal comes along. The bottom line is, if neurotransmitter levels are out of balance, so is your mood and sense of well-being.

The solution? Rebalance your brain biochemistry so your brain neurotransmitter levels are optimized. Since I've been emphasizing the importance of neurotransmitters, it's time to discuss what makes them so special when it comes to depression.

## A PRIMER ON NEUROTRANSMITTERS

Most neurotransmitters are made from amino acids, which are the building blocks of proteins. Because you get your protein from food, it follows that a diet deficient in protein would also be lacking in amino acids, leaving your body unable to produce enough neurotransmitters to keep your brain functioning in top form and to keep depression at arm's length. The primary neurotransmitters associated with depression and related mood disorders are the following:

• **Serotonin.** This is the neurotransmitter most people recognize by name and most often associate with depression, largely because it is the one targeted by many of today's antidepressant drugs. Serotonin is one of the main stimulators of the pleasure centers in the brain, so when levels in the brain are sufficient, you are likely to feel relaxed, confident, secure, and emotionally stable. Low levels are associated with depression as well as anxiety, insomnia, obsessive-compulsive behaviors, and cravings for sugar and carbohydrates.

• **GABA (gamma aminobutyric acid).** This neurotransmitter is found in both the brain and the spinal cord. It is similar to serotonin in that it helps to inhibit the transmission of electrical signals between neurons (see "Two Types of Neurotransmitters" on page 10). It is manufactured in the body from the amino acid glutamate, with the help of vitamins C and $B_6$. Using sophisticated proton magnetic resonance spectroscopy, researchers have been able to see that concentrations of GABA are reduced in the brain, plasma, and cerebrospinal fluid in people who are depressed when compared with controls.

• **Dopamine.** Like serotonin, dopamine is a major stimulator of the pleasure centers in the brain. In fact, researchers have tracked the activity of dopamine in the brain to areas known to promote feelings of satisfaction, euphoria, and sexual pleasure. Low levels can cause apathy, irritability, and a tendency to be addicted to alcohol or other recreational drugs.

• **Norepinephrine** (also called noradrenaline). This neurotransmitter plays a role in how your body responds to stress and anxiety—your fight-or-flight reaction to physical danger or a perceived sense of harm. When you are faced with a threat, norepinephrine acts on the nerves that control your blood pressure, heart rate, and breathing, and has a role in how quickly the sugar in your bloodstream can be converted into energy. When norepinephrine levels are adequate, you feel alert, positive, and full of energy. Low levels of norepinephrine activity in the brain are associated with depression, fatigue, apathy, reduced sex drive, and difficulty focusing and concentrating.

• **Epinephrine** (also called adrenaline). Like norepinephrine, epinephrine is involved in how your body responds to stressful situations. It is similar to norepinephrine in other respects as well. The adrenal medulla produces epinephrine, and both it and norepinephrine are produced from dopamine. All three neurotransmitters are excitatory (see "Two Types of Neurotransmitters" on page 10).

• **Glutamate.** This neurotransmitter also has an excitatory role when it comes to mood, and is the most prevalent and main excitatory neurotransmitter in the brain. Excessive glutamate activity is associated with anxiety and agitation. High levels in the brain are associated with behavioral problems in children.

• **Glutamine.** Although technically not a neurotransmitter, glutamine plays an extremely important role in the brain. One of its functions is to facilitate the brain's use of glucose, which is this organ's main source of fuel. It is the only compound other than glucose that may be used as fuel in the brain. Glutamine also regulates the brain's level of ammonia, which has a positive effect on mood and energy level. A deficiency of glutamine is characterized by a craving for sugary foods, a low sex drive, and a tendency toward alcohol abuse.

*These neurotransmitters, and the specific amino acids that you can take as food and/or supplements to promote their production, are key components in my treatment approach to depression*, so you can expect to read a lot more about them throughout this book. I also discuss other neurotransmitters that play a lesser but still influential role in mood, including histamine, glycine, glutamic acid, phenylethylamine (PEA), and acetylcholine.

## Two Types of Neurotransmitters

Neurotransmitters can be divided into two groups: inhibitory and excitatory. These two types of neurotransmitters work together to ensure that important signals are transmitted and unimportant ones are not.

• **Inhibitory.** Serotonin and GABA are primarily inhibitory, which means they have the ability to suppress the signal-sending activity of neurons. (Under certain circumstances, serotonin can be stimulatory.) GABA is the primary inhibitory neurotransmitter, and it inhibits excitatory neurotransmitters when they are overactive; an elevation of GABA activity is generally a response to such overactivity.

• **Excitatory.** Dopamine, norepinephrine, epinephrine, and glutamate are excitatory, which means they can make certain neurons more likely to generate an electrical signal. Glutamate is the primary stimulatory neurotransmitter, and epinephrine, norepinephrine, and dopamine tend to modulate glutamate activity.

Without getting into the complexities of how and why

these two types of neurotransmitters work in the brain, let's just say that the reason it is important to know the difference between these two types is that *effective treatment of depression depends on starting to balance the inhibitory neurotransmitters, then balancing the excitatory neurotransmitter levels, and then maintaining a balance between the two.* To attempt treatment in reverse order may result in unpleasant side effects, such as anxiety and agitation. Therefore, I always identify which neurotransmitters appear to be out of balance (using a process I explain in chapter 3), and then take steps to correct the inhibitory levels and then the excitatory levels using orthomolecular and other natural approaches to achieve and maintain optimal brain biochemistry.

Now that you better understand why neurotransmitters are so instrumental in depression, let's consider other factors that contribute to depression. As you review these factors, keep in mind that all interact with each other, often contributing to neurotransmitter imbalances.

## OTHER CAUSES OF DEPRESSION

It's become evident in recent years that depression is a complex condition and that there are many contributing factors to consider. These factors include:

- Nutritional imbalances.
- Hormonal imbalances.
- Exposure to toxic substances.
- An unhealthy balance among the gastrointestinal tract, immune system, and nervous system, including food reactions.

- Inadequate exposure to sunlight.
- Chronic disease.
- Medication use.
- Genetics and gender.

Unfortunately, most conventional health-care practitioners ignore or give superficial attention to these considerations. The encouraging news is that like neurotransmitter imbalances, the issues we discuss here—even genetics—can be changed, meaning that you have the power to improve or eliminate them as contributors to or causes of your depressed mood. The more causes you can identify and correct, the more positive, self-confident, and balanced you will feel.

## Nutritional Imbalances

The standard American diet (SAD) lives up to its name: nutritionally poor and calorie-rich, it leaves many people overfed but poorly nourished. The impact of diet on mood is very significant and somewhat complex. Nutritional imbalances are also clearly associated with neurotransmitters and amino acids, so it is easy to see how correcting all of these imbalances is a critical part of my treatment program. I have therefore dedicated a separate chapter to how food influences mood (see chapter 2).

## Hormonal Imbalances

Along with neurotransmitters, hormones also top the list of substances that play a critical role in determining how we feel and act. In fact, *neurotransmitters and hormones function as a unit, so when one or more neurotransmitters are out of balance, it's very likely that one or more hormones will be as well.* This is important to remember, because for many people it is necessary to adopt treatment strategies that will bring elements in both areas back into balance. *Conventional antidepressant drug therapy does not address this issue; an orthomolecular/natural approach does.*

Endocrine glands (including the pituitary, thyroid, pineal, adrenals, ovaries, and testes) produce chemicals called *hormones* that they release into the bloodstream to regulate the development and activities of targeted tissues throughout the body. Some hormones are manufactured in the brain as well. Whenever there is a malfunction anywhere in the production process—either too much or too little of a hormone is made—a hormonal imbalance occurs, and depression may be a consequence.

Of the dozens of hormones the body produces, we will concern ourselves with the ones that have the most significant effect on mood: cortisol (stress hormone), sex hormones (estrogen, progesterone, and testosterone), thyroid hormones, dehydroepiandrosterone (DHEA), pregnenolone, and melatonin, all of which are explored in detail in chapter 9.

## Exposure to Toxins

Modern society's insatiable desire for bigger, faster, and more "stuff" has brought us many conveniences, but the unfortunate side effects have been the creation and deposition of toxins, including heavy metals and agricultural, industrial, and household chemicals, that can have a detrimental effect on emotional and physical health. These toxins are everywhere: in food, in the air, in the soil, and in the products we use every day, such as the furniture in our homes, paint on the walls, carpeting on the floor, paper in the copier, and medications we take.

Toxins that directly affect the nervous system are called *neurotoxins.* Since the nervous system is closely connected to the immune and endocrine systems, neurotoxins affect their functions as well. Neurotoxins such as lead, mercury, formaldehyde, dioxins, and thousands of other poisons in the environment can build up gradually in the body and cause symptoms of toxicity including depression, fatigue, lethargy, headache, nervousness, sudden anger, memory loss, and a predisposition to chronic infection.

In chapter 8, I will be discussing the toxic heavy metals or minerals (arsenic, aluminum, cadmium, lead, and mercury) as well as other toxic substances, such as fluoride and organic toxins. I will explain how to avoid them and how to remove them once they are present in the body. For many patients, detoxifying plays an important role in reducing depression and other symptoms.

## The Gut, Immune System, and Nervous System

If you always thought depression was in your head, consider this: It may actually start in your gut (intestinal tract). If the mucosal lining of the gut has been damaged by prolonged use of medication or alcohol, or because of a condition that compromises the intestinal wall such as celiac disease, candidiasis, or hypothyroidism, *leaky gut* can develop. In leaky gut, the intestinal lining is abnormally permeable to large molecules and other damaging substances, including toxins and antigens.

These molecules pass through the gut wall, enter the bloodstream, and are carried to different parts of the body, including the brain, where they can affect the function of neurons and neurotransmitters. When the molecules that leave the gut and enter the bloodstream include undigested food molecules, the result can be a food reaction—"brain sensitivity"—either because of a direct effect or because the immune system considers these molecules to be foreign invaders and so attacks them, which in turn affects the nervous system and affects mood. Some of these large molecules can pass into the bloodstream, bind to opioid receptors in the brain, and cause abnormal behavior. (See chapter 2 for more on leaky gut.)

## Food Reactions

Back in the early 1980s, my late colleague Dr. David Sheinkin and I teamed up with writer Richard Hutton to write a book titled *Food, Mind and Mood*, which discusses concepts that are still relevant today. Among them is the fact that in some people, certain foods cause various reactions, including depression, gastrointestinal problems, and rash. Among orthomolecular psychiatrists, naturopaths, clinical ecologists, and specialists in environmental medicine, there is a consensus that "allergies" can affect not only the skin, respiratory system, or digestive tract, but also the brain. These types of allergies are called brain allergies or allergies of the nervous system. Depression is a common sympton of brain allergy, but others, such as attention deficit hyperactivity disorder (ADHD) in children, may occur as well.

Food reactions can be divided into three main categories. All three types can be helped using special diets, which I discuss in chapter 7.

- **Food allergies.** This type of food reaction occurs when the immune system reacts to a specific food by creating immunoglobulin E (IgE) antibodies. When these antibodies react with the food, the body sends out histamine and other chemicals, which can stimulate reactions such as hives, breathing problems, or stomach upset. These reactions generally remain throughout your life. Once you have this type of reaction to shrimp, for example, you always will.

- **Delayed food reactions.** This reaction also involves the immune system, but immunoglobulin G (IgG) antibodies are produced. Symptoms can take up to three days to appear. Many patients find that adopting one of the special diets is the most effective thing they can do to improve their mood and associated symptoms.

- **Food intolerances.** These reactions do *not* involve the immune system, but are characterized by reactions that can be similar to those caused by a food allergy. This group includes lactase deficiency, which leads to lactose intolerance and symptoms such as gas, cramps, and bloating. Other examples include an inability to break down gluten and casein because of an enzyme deficiency. The lack of the proper enzymes results in the accumulation of poorly digested peptides that can enter the bloodstream because of a leaky gut (see chapter 2) and be transported to the brain, where they can cause various neurological symptoms. The undigested food can also nurture abnormal bacteria or yeast in the colon. These organisms may produce toxic substances that get into the bloodstream, travel to the brain, and cause depression or other symptoms.

## Inadequate Sunlight

For many people, more than 90 percent of their supply of vitamin D comes from exposure to the sun's ultraviolet B rays. Thus, insufficient sun exposure can result in a vitamin D deficiency. This is critical, because there are definite connections among sunlight, vitamin D, and depression. A type of depression usually associated with insufficient sun exposure and a vitamin D deficiency is seasonal affective disorder (SAD), which I discuss in chapter 3. At the same time, lack of sunlight disrupts the production of melatonin, a hormone that regulates the sleep–wake cycle, by the pineal gland. Both light therapy and vitamin D are highly effective in alleviating SAD (see chapters 3, 6, and 10).

## Chronic Disease

Millions of people have chronic physical conditions that take a continuing toll on their body and emotions. Such conditions include diabetes, Parkinson's disease, heart disease, and others. These conditions frequently cause or contribute to depression.

Which came first, the depression or the condition? Increasing evidence indicates that depression can be a risk factor for these diseases *as well as a result of them.* For example, as part of the Women's Health Initiative, researchers found that subclinical depression, which most doctors fail to identify in their patients, may increase the risk of cardiovascular disease among women ages fifty to seventy. Another study, in which patients were studied for forty years, found that people with a history of clinical depression were twice as likely to develop coronary artery disease. In some cases, depression appears to result from biological effects of chronic conditions, especially those affecting the central nervous system (such as Parkinson's disease and cerebrovascular disease) and endocrine disorders (like hypothyroidism). The American Association of Clinical Endocrinologists, for example, believes that physical causes of depression are so common that "the diagnosis of subclinical [one without obvious signs] or clinical hypothyroidism must be considered in every patient with depression." And in the mid-1980s, researchers estimated that up to 50 percent of depressed individuals have a physical condition that is either the main cause of their depression or a major contributor.

More than a hundred physical conditions can cause or contribute to a depressive state or other psychiatric disorders. Too often, a patient will present with depressive symptoms caused by another medical illness that is missed. I have chosen to discuss four conditions I believe can be significant causes of depression, yet are often overlooked. It is important to maintain a high index of suspicion for an underlying medical problem or the possibility that a medication could be causing or contributing to the depression.

## Lyme Disease

One of the most commonly underdiagnosed conditions strongly linked to depression is Lyme disease, which is transmitted to humans via a bite from a deer tick that has been infected with the bacterium *Borrelia burgdorferi*. The classic signs and symptoms of the disease, which include a bull's-eye rash, joint swelling, and flu-like symptoms (fever, tiredness, headache, and stiff neck), do not appear in many people after they have been bitten, so they do not know they have the disease. Eventually, some people may begin to experience depression, mood swings, short-term memory loss, panic attacks, and difficulty with attention.

Although more than twenty-three thousand cases of Lyme disease were reported to the Centers for Disease Control and Prevention (CDC) in 2002, some experts believe the actual numbers are much higher. Joseph J. Burrascano Jr., MD, an authority on Lyme disease, has reported that the commonly used tests for the disease have about a 30 percent false-negative rate, which means about 30 percent of people with Lyme disease may have been told they don't have the disease because their test results were negative. The longer you have Lyme disease, the worse your symptoms and the more likely you are to test negative because the infectious organisms may actually prevent the body's immune system from making the substances (antibodies) that are necessary for the positive test.

Diagnosis of Lyme disease is challenging: The disease needs to be distinguished from depression, as well as chronic fatigue syndrome, arthritis, fibromyalgia, and similar conditions. Fortunately, the results of brain scans and neuropsychological testing can help doctors determine whether symptoms relate to a psychiatric problem or Lyme disease, but this presumes they consider Lyme disease as a possible cause of depression. It is important to detect Lyme disease early in its course, when it can be treated successfully with antibiotics. A delay may cause the infection to become chronic and more difficult to treat. However, depression in patients with Lyme disease often improves with antibiotics and measures to improve immune functioning.

## Candidiasis

Candidiasis is a type of yeast infection that is the result of an overgrowth of a yeast-like organism called *Candida albicans* in the gut. In addition to being a cause of leaky gut syndrome, candidiasis is itself a condition characterized by depression. Other symptoms include fatigue, recurrent yeast infections, insomnia, poor memory, muscle aches, joint pain, and gastrointestinal complaints such as bloating and nausea.

Research shows a strong link between *Candida albicans* overgrowth and depression in individuals, especially women, who have a history of any of the following:

- Use of antibiotics, especially long-term use. Such use is common among women because antibiotics are often prescribed to treat urinary tract infections.
- Use of birth control pills.
- Recurring or persistent vaginal yeast infections.
- Recurring or persistent digestive problems.
- Use of steroids.
- Excessive ingestion of sugar and other refined carbohydrates.

Antibiotics, for example, kill bacteria indiscriminately throughout the body. This includes "good" bacteria, many of which reside in your gastrointestinal tract and perform healthful functions. Yet antibiotics do not kill yeasts, which also live in your intestinal tract, so the destruction of good bacteria leaves a bacteria-to-yeast imbalance in the gut. As this imbalance worsens, the mucosal lining of your intestines weakens. The growing yeast population sends out signals resulting in cravings for carbohydrates, including sugary foods. The more carbohydrates you eat, the more the yeast grows and the more the gut lining becomes compromised; leaky gut syndrome develops. Once this occurs, food allergens and toxins can penetrate your intestinal lining and affect your immune and nervous systems.

Candida itself also produces dozens of toxins, one of which is acetaldehyde. When acetaldehyde meets up with the neurotransmitter dopamine, it can cause depression, anxiety, poor concentration, and a "spacey" feeling. Yeast in the gut of some patients actually produces alcohol; a person might become drunk without ever drinking alcoholic beverages. Once the yeast is controlled, the person becomes sober.

If you are depressed and this candidiasis story rings true for you, treatment consisting of a special diet, nutritional supplements, and possibly anti-*Candida* medication (oral nystatin, amphotericin B, Diflucan, or others) should be considered as a therapeutic trial, since no definitive laboratory test is available at present. Left untreated, candidiasis can lead to a vicious cycle of depression and illness.

## Chronic Fatigue and Immune Dysfunction Syndrome

An estimated one to four million Americans suffer severe, often debilitating fatigue as well as depression as part of a syndrome known as chronic fatigue and immune dysfunction syndrome, or CFIDS. Other symptoms of CFIDS include visual disturbances (blurriness, sensitivity to light), chills, shortness of breath, dizziness, bowel problems (diarrhea, constipation, gas), night sweats, low-grade fever, numbness or tingling, sensitivity to heat and/or cold, rash, ringing in the ears, irregular heartbeat, dry mouth, seizures, muscle twitching, and menstrual problems.

Scientific research on the syndrome is limited and some physicians will not acknowledge that CFIDS exists, which means many people are not being diagnosed. Diagnosing

CFIDS also can be challenging, because it shares many symptoms with a number of other chronic conditions, including celiac disease, diabetes, fibromyalgia, Lyme disease, lupus, and hypothyroidism, to name a few.

Although the exact cause of CFIDS is not known, some likely candidates include:

- Assaults to the immune system by toxins, including chemicals and heavy metals, which can damage the cells and organs.
- Physical and emotional stress, which can weaken the immune system.
- Microorganisms, such as viruses (Epstein-Barr virus, herpesvirus-6) or cell wall deficient bacteria (mycoplasma).

Successfully treating CFIDS will clear depressive symptoms.

## Heart Disease

The relationship between heart disease and depression is a two-way street: Having disease leads to high rates of depression, and depression itself influences the disease and recovery from it. For example, research shows that depression alone increases the risk of dying from heart disease by 400 percent in the six months following a heart attack. That's because stress causes physical changes in the heart that deprive it of oxygen. Depression is also a typical response among people who have heart disease and is a predictor of how well they will do after having a heart attack, angina, or bypass surgery. Depression in patients with heart disease should be addressed by evaluating neurotransmitters and many of the other variables discussed in this book, and treating them accordingly.

## Medication Use

"So you're telling me, Doctor, that the very drugs I'm taking to make me feel better are actually making me feel worse?" Teresa, a fifty-one-year-old mother of two teenage boys and a part-time librarian, was sitting in my office holding two bottles in her hand: one a prescription cholesterol-lowering drug she had been taking for a year, and the other an over-the-counter ibuprofen, which she took regularly for arthritis. Teresa had been experiencing depression, fatigue, and low sexual desire for about nine months. Our evaluation showed that she had a biochemical imbalance, likely partly caused by chronic use of the medications. We instituted a program that included dietary changes, supplementation with amino acids and nutrients, and exercise that not only alleviated her depression and restored her physical and sexual energy but also allowed her to stop taking her medications (with her primary doctor's knowledge).

More than one hundred prescription, over-the-counter, and illicit drugs have the potential to cause or worsen depression, anxiety, and/or mania. Always suspect the possibility that a prescription or over-the-counter medication is causing or contributing to your depression, whether or not depression is listed as an adverse side effect. Discuss with your physician the possibility of changing your medication.

## Genetics and Gender

Do you have the genes that predispose you to depression? To answer this question, it is important to understand that there is no such thing as an absolute genetic disease: Genetics must always be considered in tandem with environment. Thus, a person whose genetics suggest a tendency toward depression (family history, for example) is not necessarily destined to be depressed. As we learn more about the genetic links to depression, we can better adjust environmental factors to reduce the likelihood that a person will become depressed.

Some twin studies, for example, indicate that the genetic risk of developing clinical depression is about 40 percent, with the remaining 60 percent due to environmental factors, including lifestyle. In the late 1980s, researchers studied the brain biochemistry of alcoholics and drug addicts. They found that certain genes produced too little of the chemicals associated with positive moods and too much of those responsible for negative moods. When the study participants were given amino acid and nutritional supplements, their mood improved significantly, and they were much more likely to avoid alcohol and drugs. In fact, the subjects who did not take the supplements were four times more likely to return to their addictive behavior.

More recently, Dr. George Zubenko, a professor of psychiatry at the University of Pittsburgh, studied the genes of people with significant depression in eighty-one families and found nineteen chromosome regions that are likely to contain genes associated with depression. Four of these regions, he discovered, were present only in women; only one was present in men alone. This suggests that more genes may help to initiate depression in women than in men, which may be one reason why more women than men may become depressed.

In fact, it's a worldwide phenomenon that women are nearly twice as likely to suffer from depression as men are. Part of the reason for this disparity may be hormonal differences (see chapter 9), but other gender-specific factors appear to play a role as well. For example, women are much more likely to experience (or have a history of) physical and/or sexual abuse and to experience other negative life situations, such as job discrimination and sexual harassment. Women also tend to ruminate or "overthink" events in their lives, and such excessive thinking can quickly develop into depression.

Men, however, tend to suppress their feelings and to express their depression by engaging in activities such as excessive drinking, drug use, overwork, or violence. Rates of alcoholism, drug abuse, and gambling are higher among men, and depression may be a reason.

Although you can't change your gender, you can change your response to the stressors in your life and take natural substances to help you. You can learn more about these approaches in part 2 of this book.

## THE CONVENTIONAL APPROACH TO TREATMENT OF DEPRESSION

Conventional psychiatrists as well as some general practitioners are most likely to prescribe drugs designed to affect one or more neurotransmitters with the hope of bringing the biochemistry of the brain back into balance. You have likely seen some of these drugs advertised on television and in magazines; or perhaps you are taking one or more of them right now. Prescribing of these drugs by health-care practitioners is done with a shotgun approach: aiming one or more drugs at the depression and hoping the drugs will blow it out of the water, so to speak, while also failing to address any of the other causes of depression we just reviewed.

Yet, as you will see in chapter 12 on psychotropic drugs, use of these medications over time actually can work *against* resolving neurotransmitter imbalances, because the medications may contribute to depletion of one or more neurotransmitters. Rather than dealing with this issue, most psychiatrists will tend to just try another medication.

Let me offer one example here of why antidepressants may fail, using the selective serotonin reuptake inhibitors (Prozac being the prototype) for illustration. SSRIs only manipulate or recycle the neurotransmitters already present; they do not trigger the body to manufacture more, which is what the body may need. An orthomolecular approach to depression, however, promotes the natural production of neurotransmitters and allows the body to heal itself.

## ORTHOMOLECULAR PSYCHIATRY AND RELATED THERAPIES

The orthomolecular psychiatry approach to depression starts out with the same concept as does the conventional approach: that depression is the result of a biochemical imbalance in the brain. Whereas conventional psychiatrists immediately try to influence this imbalance by prescribing medications, I and other orthomolecular psychiatrists, as well as other orthomolecular-oriented practitioners, conduct various biochemical tests to help us identify what those imbalances are. We then try to correct them primarily with lifestyle changes and natural substances, using medications only if the natural substances don't do the job. In orthomolecular psychiatry, we look for imbalances in the following areas:

- Neurotransmitters and related brain chemicals, which include serotonin, GABA, dopamine, epinephrine, norepinephrine, glutamine, and endorphins. *One of the main ways we correct any of these imbalances is with the use of amino acids—as nutritional supplements and/or as elements of protein in foods.* This is discussed in depth in chapters 4 and 7.

- Bionutrients, including but not limited to the B vitamins, vitamin C, essential fatty acids, zinc, and others, as well as herbs. In this category, I consider dietary intake and supplementation as courses of treatment. Discussion of this approach is in chapters 5, 6, and 7.

- Hormones, including melatonin, DHEA, thyroid hormones, cortisol, progesterone, estrogen, testosterone, and adrenaline. A detailed look at hormone balancing appears in chapter 9.

As you can see, rather than aiming to change the levels of one or two neurotransmitters with drugs—and often missing!—an orthomolecular approach considers the cause of any imbalances that can have an impact on mood and then provides the body with natural substances in amounts sufficient to correct them.

## Beyond Orthomolecular Psychiatry

Treating depression with amino acid therapy, proper diet, supplementation (with nutrients, herbs, and other natural substances), and adjustment of hormone levels are all critical, effective ways to achieve your depression-free goal. However, as our discussion of the "Other Causes of Depression" shows, there are more factors to be considered. Factors that are largely ignored by conventional medicine and psychiatry but can be very important are therefore addressed in this book. These include:

- The need for adequate exposure to sunlight. We often hear about the dangers of too much sun exposure, but a safe and necessary amount of sunlight exposure helps ward off depression, as does a light box (discussed in chapters 6 and 10).
- The identification and treatment of chronic disease, as discussed earlier.
- The maintenance of healthy relationships among the brain, the gastrointestinal (GI) tract, and the immune and nervous systems. These three systems have an intimate bond (discussed in chapter 2).
- The adoption of a positive lifestyle, including adequate sleep and exercise, stress reduction and management, and mind–body work (discussed in chapter 10).
- Energy balancing, through use of acupuncture, homeopathy, and other energy medicines (discussed in chapter 11).

## THE BOTTOM LINE

Depression can be treated successfully and safely, often without the use of drugs, *if* you allow your body to heal itself by giving it the natural ingredients it needs to do so. Successful treatment of depression is about being good to you on all levels—physically, mentally, emotionally, and spiritually—and therefore requires a multifaceted approach.

## Chapter 2

_Why Are You Depressed?
You Are What You Eat_

When I say the words _comfort food,_ what comes to mind? Perhaps you are envisioning a bowl of pasta; or you may be salivating over the image of ice cream, potato chips, and, everyone's favorite, chocolate. If it sometimes seems that eating a bowl of chocolate chip ice cream improves your mood, this feeling is not just in your head. _Food_ does _affect your mood. What you eat, and when you eat it, can have a significant impact on depression._ In this chapter, you'll learn about how food influences mood.

Consider Sandra, a thirty-four-year-old junior account executive who came to me complaining of depression, fatigue, irritability, mood swings, and an inability to concentrate. Sandra had her eye on moving up the corporate ladder, and so she was worried that these problems would prevent her from moving forward in her field.

During her initial intake interview at my Center, which included a meeting with a nutritionist as standard procedure,

Sandra talked about her eating habits, and they were quite revealing. Her breakfast, if she had it, typically consisted of a
doughnut and coffee she picked up at a drive-through window
on her way to work. Sandra is a self-proclaimed lover of java,
and she admitted to consuming at least four to five cups per
day. Lunch would vary, depending on whether she had a
luncheon meeting or not, but she tended to order burgers,
fried shrimp, french fries, and other foods "I know aren't good
for me." On days when she didn't have a meeting, she might
have a microwavable dried soup or buy fries and a diet soda.
Dinner, which she sometimes ate as late as 11 PM after working late, usually consisted of microwavable pizza or a burrito,
which she washed down with a soft drink. If she was too tired
to tackle the microwave, she ate ice cream.

With nary a fruit or vegetable in sight, Sandra ate and
drank plenty of stimulants (sugar, caffeine) and processed
foods. Sandra's diet was clearly nutrient-deficient and a prime
example of one that supports depression and fatigue. To make
a long story short, we conducted a few tests and found nutritional deficiencies, determined that she was depleted in serotonin, and started her on a few amino acids (see chapter 4), a
selected supplement plan (chapter 6), some vitamin and mineral injections to kick-start her recovery, and a healthy eating
program (chapter 7). Within a week of starting this regimen,
Sandra said she felt somewhat better emotionally and physically. She became convinced that she was on the right track.
Within one month, Sandra said she felt like a new person—
she wasn't depressed, her moods had stabilized, she had lots of
energy, and she felt confident at work. She even noticed that
her relationships with her clients had improved. All this was
achieved without the use of drugs.

Can a change in diet really have a significant impact on depression? You bet it can. In this chapter, I talk about how many Americans are eating themselves into depression: how nutrient-deficient, free-radical-rich, high-calorie diets both cause and contribute to depressed mood. I will also discuss how low-calorie diets, missed meals, and other "dieting" strategies can quickly deplete the body of nutrients necessary to maintain biochemical balance and balanced mood.

## YOU ARE WHAT YOU EAT AND PROCESS

How diet affects health was dramatically demonstrated in the 2004 movie *Super Size Me*. The filmmaker filmed himself while eating nothing but fast food from McDonald's for a month. To the surprise of physicians who agreed to follow him during this time, not only did his mood change drastically, but he almost died of liver failure as a result of damage from this diet. All in only one month! It is clear that *most* of the foods you eat play a role in your mood and your health. But the old adage "You are what you eat" needs to be modified to "You are what you eat, digest, absorb, and assimilate." In the following sections, we'll examine the digestive process, potential digestive problems, and how your choice of foods can affect your health and your mood.

### The Digestive Process, Digestive Enzymes, and Leaky Gut

Eating nutritious food is essential for good health, but if your digestive system isn't operating optimally, you will cheat your body of well-deserved and much-needed nutrients that can significantly impact your mood. Digestion starts in the mouth, where ideally you should chew your food until it is reduced to liquid before you swallow it. Chewing is accompanied by the release of saliva from the salivary glands. The saliva contains enzymes, including amylase, lingual lipase, and ptyalin, which begin the process of digesting fats and starches.

The food then passes through the esophagus into the stomach, where hydrochloric acid, mucus, and proteolytic enzymes are secreted to act on the food. Hydrochloric acid stimulates pepsinogen to form pepsin, an enzyme that helps to break down proteins into smaller peptide molecules (*polypeptides*), and gastric lipase, which helps to break down fats. The acidic environment of the stomach helps destroy disease-causing microorganisms that may enter the stomach with the food. If, however, stomach acid production is impaired, organisms such as *Candida* or *Helicobacter pylori* can reproduce and cause stomach inflammation and depressive symptoms. In addition, a deficiency of stomach acid can cause poor breakdown of proteins, which leads to poor absorption of amino acids and a negative effect on mood. The extremely widespread use of stomach antacids and acid blocker medication significantly contributes to many people having inadequate acid in their stomachs for proper gastric digestion.

In a healthy gut, the digested food then passes into the small intestine, where further digestion occurs and where most of the nutrients are absorbed into the bloodstream. Ideally, the pancreas secretes bicarbonate and other enzymes into the small intestine, and the small intestine also secretes enzymes to further break down food particles. With the help of bile formed in the liver and secreted into the small intestine to help break down fats, the smallest food particles are absorbed into the circulation for use everywhere in the body.

When the breakdown of food is incomplete, problems may occur. For example, some polypeptides have properties similar to endorphins (neurotransmitters that have painkilling properties and are involved in determining mood) and are called *exorphins*. These exorphins, which are large molecules of protein fragments, are formed from incomplete digestion of gluten (found in wheat and other grains) and casein (found in milk), two substances that cause food reactions in some people. I discuss gluten and casein and their exorphins in chapter 7. In people who have a healthy gut, exorphins and other large molecules cannot escape the intestinal tract and are further broken down by the digestive enzymes (such as trypsin and chymotrypsin) before they are absorbed into the bloodstream. For this process to occur properly, a person needs to have sufficient hydrochloric acid in the stomach to help enzymes there start protein digestion; sufficient enzymes and bicarbonate in the small intestine to continue the digestive process; and a relatively undamaged small intestinal lining, which serves as a filter to allow nutritive substances into the bloodstream and prevent larger, potentially damaging molecules (like exorphins) from entering the bloodstream. If large molecules do get through the intestinal barrier, the individual has increased intestinal permeability, or leaky gut.

The small intestine leads into the large intestine, or colon, *which harbors more bacteria—healthful and harmful—than all of the cells of the body.* Thus, the health of the large intestine holds a key to your overall health, which is why I stress the importance of intestinal health. The colon is also where fluid is reabsorbed into the bloodstream and feces are formed. Feces are moved through the colon via muscular contractions and eventually exit the body through the anus. Feces also are a vehicle through which toxins that are processed by the liver for detoxification can leave the body.

## Digestive Enzymes

The primary digestive enzymes in the body are proteases (which digest proteins), amylases (which digest carbohydrates), and lipases (which digest fats). Bile produced in the liver and secreted into the small intestine helps break down fats. The pancreas produces most of the digestive enzymes, but other sites along the digestive tract (such as the salivary glands, stomach, and small intestine) produce enzymes as well. Inadequate enzyme reserves in the body can result from a variety of situations, including caffeine and alcohol consumption, illness, pregnancy, stress, and aging, because there is a decline in digestive enzyme secretion with age.

The main reason for a deficiency of digestive enzymes is the poor diet that many Americans follow: It contains fewer raw foods (good sources of enzymes) than it once did, and many more processed foods, which contain virtually no enzymes. Foreign chemicals in the food (such as preservatives and other artificial chemicals) may interfere with proper enzyme function. Cooking also destroys naturally occurring enzymes. An enzyme deficiency leads to poor digestion and poor absorption of nutrients, which in turn can result in food reactions, overgrowth of unfriendly bacteria and yeast, indigestion, constipation, bloating, headaches, fatigue, and other problems. To help prevent or eliminate a digestive enzyme deficiency, eat a more healthful diet and consider taking digestive enzyme supplements. Both of these topics are discussed in chapter 7.

## WHAT YOU EAT

Now let's look at the food you eat. As you go through this section, make note of the types of foods you typically consume each day. Are the foods you eat most often ones that promote or support a good mood, or those that tend to fuel depression?

### Protein

Protein is a *macronutrient* (needed in relatively large amounts, as opposed to *micronutrients*, which are needed in only small amounts) and the primary building material of the body's tissues. It also has other functions: It helps balance hormone and blood sugar levels (also important in depression, as you will learn in subsequent chapters), heal wounds, control sugar cravings, and strengthen the immune system. In addition, it has a significant impact on mood and mental functioning, because it is composed of substances called amino acids, which have a direct effect on the levels and activities of certain brain chemicals, including neurotransmitters and endorphins.

Unless you consume an adequate amount of protein every day, your brain will not be able to manufacture sufficient levels of the mood-enhancing neurotransmitters it needs. How much protein do you need? Each person's protein needs are different, but generally, you should consume at least 2 ounces of high-quality protein three times a day, at each meal. The generally accepted protein requirement is 0.8 gram per kilogram (2.2 pounds). However, some people find that they function better on considerably more protein. If you are protein-deficient and add sufficient protein to your daily intake, you will likely experience an improvement in mood within just a few weeks.

I want to make clear that protein in food is broken down in the digestive tract to form amino acids, which are absorbed into the bloodstream. The amino acids are then used by the body to make its own proteins, as well as the smaller-molecule neurotransmitters. Although the body manufactures protein from twenty amino acids, only seven of them appear to play a significant role in depression: tryptophan, phenylalanine, 5-hydroxytryptophan (5-HTP), tyrosine, glutamine, gamma aminobutyric acid (GABA), and S-adenosylmethionine (SAMe, a metabolite of the amino acid methionine; it is discussed at the beginning of part 2 of this book, relating to methylation). I revisit these amino acids in depth in chapter 4. For now, you should know that all the amino acids need some assistance if they are to work optimally in your body. That's where complex carbohydrates come into the picture.

## Complex Carbohydrates

Carbohydrates are the sugar and starch components of food and consist of hydrogen, carbon, and oxygen. Sugars are simple carbohydrates—they consist of a single molecule or two molecules chained together—while starches consist of multiple sugars bound together. Examples of sugars are body sugar (glucose), fruit sugar (fructose), milk sugar (lactose), and table sugar (sucrose). Glucose and fructose are single molecules, while sucrose and lactose consist of two sugar molecules bound together to form one molecule.

Carbohydrates play a major role in energy production in the body. When sugar is burned or oxidized (combined with oxygen), it forms adenosine triphosphate (ATP). ATP molecules provide energy for most of the biochemical reactions that occur in the body. Another very important function of certain sugars is to combine with proteins (a combination called a glycoprotein) to allow for cell-to-cell communication within the body. This communication is necessary for many functions, including immune functioning and brain cell communication. We discuss the role of these essential sugars in more detail in chapter 7.

Carbohydrates can also be either refined or unrefined. We find unrefined carbohydrates in whole foods, such as whole grains, fruits, and vegetables. These foods contain not only starch and/or sugar, but also fiber, vitamins, minerals, and other nutrients. In refined carbohydrates, the fiber is removed, along with a variety of nutrients. White bread and white refined sugar are common examples of refined carbohydrates. These refined carbohydrates are often referred to as empty calories because they contain the calories but not the nutrients or fiber present in the unrefined carbohydrates. Their nutrient density is very poor.

Unlike simple carbohydrates, which the body metabolizes rapidly, thus providing a quick "high" followed by a quick low, complex carbohydrates provide a more steady supply of energy. Complex carbohydrates also are instrumental in improving mood, and here's why.

When you eat complex carbohydrates along with foods rich in tryptophan, the carbohydrates help tryptophan to enter the brain to form serotonin, a neurotransmitter that is frequently low in depressed patients. For example, say you've just eaten a meal rich in protein. Your stomach and intestine break down the protein to its component amino acids. The amino acids travel in the bloodstream to various tissues, including muscles and the brain. When the amino acids reach the brain, they compete with each other to get into the brain, and their rate of entry is limited. Thus, if many amino acids are present, the entrance of tryptophan into the brain will be slow and limited. Carbohydrates help get tryptophan into the brain by diverting the other amino acids into muscles, thus reducing tryptophan's competition for entering the brain.

The proposed mechanism for this is as follows: As complex carbohydrates break down and release glucose (body sugar), the glucose stimulates the pancreas to secrete insulin. One of the main functions of insulin is to help glucose into cells where it is used to produce energy; another is to help the amino acids in your bloodstream get into your muscle cells. However, although insulin allows almost all amino acids entry into cells, it does not do this for tryptophan. By enabling the other amino acids to enter the muscle cells, insulin reduces the nontryptophan amino acids in the bloodstream, thus reducing the competition for tryptophan getting into the brain to produce serotonin. Most fruits and vegetables, whole grains and whole-grain products (including brown rice), dried beans, and legumes boost serotonin levels in this way.

## Refined Carbohydrates

Americans love sugar. In 1900, the average American consumed 25 pounds of sugar a year. By the 1990s, consumption had increased more than fivefold to surpass 125 pounds of sugar per person. Regular consumption of refined sugars and starches has a detrimental effect on neurotransmitter activity in the brain. The main ingredients in many popular foods such as doughnuts, cakes, cookies, Danish, breakfast cereals, and pies are sugar and starch. Sugar is the main ingredient in nondiet sodas, and starch is the main ingredient in white bread, bagels, and pasta. These are the types of foods with which millions of Americans start their day, and continue to eat throughout the day as temporary energy boosters.

Here's how sugar works. Carbohydrates increase the level of tryptophan, a precursor to the neurotransmitter serotonin, in the blood. Within minutes of eating carbohydrates, serotonin levels rise. Unlike complex carbohydrates, however, refined carbohydrates enter the bloodstream quickly and decline quickly. Tryptophan and serotonin levels rise rapidly but then fall quickly. As levels of neurotransmitters decline, so does mood. Yet you still crave simple carbohydrates, because, as you may have experienced, these foods have a drug-like (comfort-food) effect. You may experience temporary calm or a brief energy boost every time you eat them, but you have become addicted to their effects.

In addition to its effects on neurotransmitters, sugar consumption also has a direct impact on blood sugar levels, which in turn affects mood. When you consume too much sugar, it goes directly into your bloodstream, and you get a "high." Your body tries to stabilize blood sugar levels, so it produces lots of insulin to move the excess sugar from the blood into cells. Often, insulin overshoots and causes blood sugar to go too low. At this point, you may feel fatigued or depressed, or have a sense of impending doom (since your brain is not getting enough fuel to function). The adrenal glands kick in to produce the fight-or-flight hormones epinephrine (adrenaline) and norepinephrine (noradrenaline), which stimulate the liver to break down starch into sugar and bring the blood sugar back to normal. At this point, you may feel shaky, anxious, or agitated from the effects of excessive epinephrine. Alternatively, or in addition, as the blood sugar level drops, you may again have the urge to eat more sugar or starch to raise your blood sugar. For many people, this roller-coaster effect occurs day after day, resulting in extreme stress to the adrenal glands (the stress glands) and continued depletion of the neurotransmitters.

## Fat

Many food manufacturers and advertisers would have you believe that fat intake is the enemy, and so for the past few years, the market has been flooded with low-fat and fat-free foods. People in droves have been buying them. Yet despite the popularity of such foods, Americans on average continue to get fatter and more depressed. Clearly, we need to have a better understanding of the role of fats in both mental and physical health and what constitutes healthful fats.

Many are surprised to learn that the brain is more than 60 percent fat. Most of this fat must come from food, so if you are eating a low-fat diet—low in the fats essential for optimal brain function—this may be playing a significant role in your depression. You do need to consume a sufficient amount of healthful fats for maximum brain function, and to avoid fats that interfere with fat metabolism and damage health. Fats have three functions in the body: They are used for energy, they are part of the structure of every cell membrane in the body, and they make local hormones that can have profound effects on the body. Essential fatty acids are necessary for two of these functions, namely to make up the cell membrane and to make the local hormones called prostaglandins. The essential fatty acids are:

- **Omega-3 fatty acids.** These are eicosapentaenoic acid

(EPA) and docosahexaenoic acid (DHA), found primarily in cold-water fish, and alpha linolenic acid (ALA), present in flaxseed and some nuts, seeds, and other plants.

• **Omega-6 fatty acids.** Those come in the form of linoleic acid, found in most vegetable oils.

I have found that *achieving and maintaining an optimal balance of these essential fatty acids is an integral part of a successful treatment program for treatment of depression.* Consuming too little healthy fat can result in low serotonin levels, which translates into low mood.

Evidence points to a relationship between the steady declines in the amount of omega-3 fatty acids Americans eat in their diets and the rise in depression. Some studies also show that populations of people who eat a large amount of fish (an excellent source of omega-3) have low rates of major depression.

And what about the omega-6 fatty acids? Americans are sometimes deficient in these essential fatty acids as well because frequently the oils containing linoleic acid have been damaged with deep-frying or through hydrogenation (see chapter 5), resulting in poorly functioning omega-6 fatty acids. We discuss the fats in more depth in chapter 5.

## Vitamins, Minerals, and Other Essential Nutrients

Besides the three macronutrients—protein, carbohydrates, and fats—you also need a variety of vitamins, minerals, and other essential nutrients, which work with and complement the activities of the macronutrients as well as neurotransmitters and hormones. The best sources of these nutrients are whole, fresh foods such as quality animal protein (beef, poultry, fish, eggs, and dairy), fruits, vegetables, whole grains, legumes, and seeds that are prepared and consumed in a form that involves little or no processing. Yet we are a fast-food nation, and convenience is the driving force. Much of the food Americans eat has been refined, processed, and packaged into time-saving morsels: drive-through-window food, microwavable dinners, frozen entrées, add-water-and-stir soups. Commercial food processing not only adds unhealthy artificial colors and flavors and preservatives to your foods but also strips foods of essential nutrients that the neurotransmitters need to function optimally. Even marginal vitamin and mineral deficiencies that don't result in clinical symptoms can have a negative effect on your mood.

The list of nutrients that can impact mood is long, and I discuss many of them in chapter 6. Here, we will look at your consumption of fresh fruits and vegetables, which are excellent sources of these nutrients. Are you eating at least five to seven servings of these foods daily, either raw or lightly steamed (not fried) to retain their nutritional value? Refer to the box to determine what constitutes a serving.

---

### Serving Size for Fruits and Vegetables

- ½ cup cooked or chopped raw fruit or vegetable
- 1 cup raw leafy vegetable
- 1 medium piece of fruit
- ¼ cup dried fruit
- 6 ounces vegetable or fruit juice

---

## Caffeine

Caffeine is on my "Foods to Avoid" list (see chapter 7), and here's why. The problem is that, like sugar, caffeine can take you on a roller-coaster ride of ups and downs during the day, and you may wind up extremely dependent on it. When you stop taking caffeine, you may experience significant withdrawal effects, including severe headaches, mood swings, and fatigue. Caffeine stimulates your nervous system and your adrenal glands, which produces stress. It's also been shown that people who drink the most coffee often experience chronic depression.

A more direct association between caffeine and depression, however, is that it inhibits the brain's levels of serotonin and the hormone into which it converts, melatonin, which aids in sleep. In addition, caffeine depletes the body of nutrients that are essential to maintaining good mood, including vitamin C, magnesium, calcium, zinc, potassium, and the B vitamins. Caffeine also hinders the normal metabolism of GABA, which is manufactured in the intestines and, like serotonin, calms stress and anxiety.

## Alcohol

Does drinking alcohol cause people to be depressed, or do people drink alcohol because they are depressed? The answer to both questions is yes. A depressed person may drink alcohol to depress some of the brain's inhibitory functions, thus reducing inhibitions and achieving a lifting of mood. Alcohol is a depressant, however, and larger amounts will tend to inhibit the excitatory functions of the brain and ultimately make the person more depressed. Alcohol consumption also reduces the body's ability to extract nutrients from food, especially the B vitamins, which play an important role in neurotransmitter production.

## Organic Versus Nonorganic Food

I advise my patients to eat organic foods whenever possible, for two reasons. First, organic foods are less likely to have harmful pesticides and other toxic substances. Second, the soil in which organic foods are grown is likely to contain more trace minerals and other nutrients that are often lacking in soil treated with conventional fertilizers; the latter contains the least amount of nutrients necessary to support growth, and many essential nutrients are lacking. As more and more people realize the benefits of organic foods and demand them, these foods will become much more readily available in mainstream supermarkets, and more affordable.

## DEPRESSION, DIETING, AND OTHER FOOD ISSUES

### Dieting, Eating Disorders, and Depression

Given that Americans spend approximately $40 billion each year on diet-related purchases—books, programs, supplements, special foods—you would hope to see a much better success rate when it comes to weight loss. Yet more than 90 percent of people who go on a diet and lose weight can expect to gain back every pound, and even a few pounds more, within a few months or years of the weight loss. And the number of overweight Americans keeps rising. According to the Centers for

Disease Control and Prevention's National Health and Nutrition Examination Survey, about 64 percent of American adults are carrying excessive pounds: 33 percent are overweight (with a body mass index [BMI] greater than 25) and 31 percent are obese (BMI greater than 30). (BMI is calculated using a formula that relates a person's height to his/her weight, with normal being in the 18.5 to 24.9 range. It is a person's weight in kilograms divided by height in meters.)

There are smart ways as well as not-so-smart ways to lose excess weight, and fasting, skipping meals, and otherwise severely restricting caloric intake are examples of the latter. There are many problems associated with this approach to weight loss—not least of which is that it rarely succeeds—but the ones we are concerned with are those associated with mood.

One of the first things that happens when people go on a low-calorie diet is that their serotonin levels decline, because typically they get little or very little tryptophan. As discussed under "Protein," tryptophan promotes serotonin production. Because few foods contain high levels of tryptophan, it is often one of the first nutrients to become depleted when people go on a low-calorie diet. The same is true for phenylalanine, which converts to dopamine, norepinephrine, and endorphins.

Low-calorie dieters also usually deprive themselves of sufficient amounts of the nutrients that are essential for preventing depression. Another effect of low-calorie dieting is a decline in thyroid function, a protective mechanism the body has developed to conserve energy when a person ingests too few calories. I discuss the role of iodine in relation to the thyroid in chapter 6 and the thyroid in relation to depression in chapter 9.

There is also a link between dieting and eating disorders.

As serotonin levels decline, feelings of self-esteem and self-confidence plummet as well. Especially among some women, the desire to be thin can become an obsession, which is actually "fed" by dieting. As these young women dramatically reduce their caloric intake in an effort to get thin, their intake of essential nutrients, including protein, also declines. When tryptophan deficiency results in a decline in serotonin levels, these individuals may get caught up in thoughts and/or behaviors they can't control. Because they are focusing on dieting and food, these dieters may become obsessed with how many calories they are consuming and eat less and less in the quest for the "perfect" body. This obsession can be the ideal stage for anorexia. Although there are usually psychological factors involved in cases of anorexia and other eating disorders, it is critical to resolve the nutritional imbalances of a starved brain in order for these individuals to heal successfully.

## Obesity and Depression

It may be too simplistic to say that obese people are depressed *because* they are overweight. What if they're obese because they're depressed? Research suggests that some obese people crave and overeat carbohydrates, literally avoiding protein foods. When obese carbohydrate cravers are asked why they eat so many high-carbohydrate foods, such as pasta and baked goods, they say they make them feel calm and in a better mood. So researchers gave carbohydrate-rich meals to people who craved carbohydrates and those who did not. Three hours after eating a high-carbohydrate meal, the cravers said they felt less depressed, but the noncravers said they felt sleepy.

People who crave carbohydrates may have a faulty "reporting" system: Their serotonin feedback system doesn't tell the brain to stop craving carbohydrates, and so their desire for them continues and they overeat. At one time, doctors prescribed drugs such as fenfluramine and Redux to increase serotonin levels in the brain and reduce appetite, but they were removed from the market because of significant side effects. A better solution for depressed carbohydrate cravers would be amino acid supplements to increase serotonin and balance the neurotransmitters.

## THE BOTTOM LINE

People are often surprised to hear that their current food choices are likely having a significant impact on their mood and that conscious changes can bring about dramatic positive results. I cannot emphasize enough the importance of balancing optimal-quality food and in the proper amounts for managing depression. Whenever possible, eat organic, unprocessed whole foods.

In these first two chapters, I introduced many different possible causes of depression. In the next chapter, I zero in on specific characteristics of those causes and offer you some tools to help you identify the possible reasons behind your depressive mood and how to treat it.

*Chapter 3*

❦

Discover Your Biochemical Profile and
Get the Professional Help You Need

$O$ne of the paradoxical things about depression is that those who suffer with it often feel too depressed to look for help. Even thinking about looking for help fills them with feelings of hopelessness. I've seen the look of despair and resignation on the faces of many men and women who have been disappointed by drug therapy, who are tired of going from doctor to doctor looking for relief, or who have simply been ready to give up. But you don't need to traipse from doctor's office to doctor's office or call it quits.

What you need is a place to start. In this chapter, I arm you with the tools you can use to begin the healing process. First, I profile the different types of depression. We are a society that likes to label everything; however, more important than labeling depression is the fact that various biochemical imbalances may cause and support your depressive symptoms. Thus, it is helpful to determine *your individual biochemical profile*, which I help you do by introducing Symptom Profiles: checklists you can use to help you identify which biochemical imbalances may be causing or contributing to your depressive mood.

Then I give a brief presentation of some of the different diagnostic tests I and other like-minded health-care practitioners use to help check for biochemical imbalances, so we can take a customized approach to treatment. In this section, I highlight the tests used to identify neurotransmitter imbalances, a new, state-of-the-art approach I have found helpful in my practice.

Next, I discuss the diagnostic process we follow at the Schachter Center for Complementary Medicine to evaluate and treat depression in a comprehensive manner. Finally, I talk about how to find professionals who can help you with your healing process.

## TYPES OF DEPRESSION AND MOOD DISORDERS

Depression is a state of being that can run the gamut from mild and temporary to severe and prolonged; from having a manageable effect on your life to throwing it into complete chaos. For some people, their mood is manageable one day but not the next.

When you are depressed, it doesn't really matter what label someone puts on your mood: You just want to feel better. Yet for research, diagnostic, and treatment purposes, experts have created classifications for depression, which should help you better understand what you are experiencing in your life.

### Major Depression

Sometimes I see an individual who clearly displays the characteristics associated with major depression, so much so that he or she could be a poster child for the condition. Liane was such a person. At thirty-eight, Liane said she felt like a woman twice her age.

"I have no energy, and I don't feel like seeing people or going out at all," she said after arriving at my office with her sister. "I wouldn't even be here if it weren't for my sister, who insisted I come."

In addition to fatigue and apathy, Liane was having a hard time concentrating and had to quit her job as a payroll clerk for a local firm. Over the past two months she had gained 20 pounds and had overwhelming feelings of worthlessness. She admitted to having recurrent thoughts of suicide and found herself sleeping twelve or more hours a night. When awake, she was usually irritable with everyone, especially family members.

Liane displayed all eight of the standard criteria for a diagnosis of major depression (see the box). Although the severity and duration of each criterion varies from person to person, to meet the definition of major depression, they must be intense enough to disrupt all facets of an individual's life.

---

### Criteria for Diagnosis of Major Depression

At any one point, 5 to 9 percent of women and 2 to 3 percent of men are suffering with major depression. Within an entire lifetime, 10 to 25 percent of women and 5 to 12 percent of men can expect to experience this condition. For a diagnosis of major depression, five or more of the following criteria must have been present during the same two-week period and represent a change from the individual's previous state of being. At least one of the symptoms must be "depressed mood" or "loss of pleasure or interest."

- Depressed mood most of the day, nearly every day, as indicated by the individual's own report or observations made by others.
- Loss of pleasure or interest in all or nearly all activities most of the day almost every day.
- Significant weight gain or loss (more than 5 percent of body weight in a month) and/or an increase or decrease in appetite nearly every day.
- Reduced ability to make decisions or concentrate almost every day.
- Fatigue or loss of energy almost every day.
- Insomnia or excessive sleeping almost every day.
- Psychomotor agitation or retardation, almost every day as observable by others.
- Feelings of excessive or inappropriate guilt and worthlessness.
- Recurring thoughts of death, suicidal ideation without a specific plan, or a suicide attempt or a specific plan to commit suicide.

## Dysthymia (Chronic Mild Depression)

If you or a loved one has experienced chronic sadness and other symptoms of depression almost daily for a long period of time, you may have dysthymia, or chronic mild depression. By some estimates, as many as forty million Americans suffer with this form of depression. The criteria for dysthymia include depressed mood that has lasted for two years for most of the day for more days than not, plus two or more of the following:

- Poor appetite or overeating.
- Insomnia or oversleeping.
- Fatigue or low energy level.
- Low self-esteem.
- Poor concentration or difficulty making decisions.
- Feeling hopeless.

These symptoms are less severe than those in people who have major depression, and many people with dysthymia enjoy periods of normal mood that last weeks or months in between their depressive episodes.

## Seasonal Affective Disorder (SAD)

For some people who live in areas that get little sunshine during the winter months, a type of depression called seasonal affective disorder may occur. It is believed to affect an estimated 5 percent of the entire US population, although the percentage may be higher in the northern New England area (about 10 percent) and lower in the southern part of the country (2 percent). Characteristics of SAD include fatigue, lethargy, sleep problems, difficulty concentrating, weight gain, and loss of interest in sex. Women are four times more likely than men to experience SAD.

The key to preventing and treating SAD is exposure to sunlight, because the condition typically strikes during sun-deprived months but disappears when the days grow longer in spring. The most popular hypothesis about SAD is that the body's natural daily rhythms are constantly adjusting themselves, and they depend on the intensity of sunlight to get cues. These cues begin in the retina in the eye and create signals to the optic nerve that travel to the brain, where they stimulate an increase in the level of serotonin, which improves mood. During this time, some serotonin converts to melatonin, which is stored in the pineal gland. At night when it is dark, the pineal gland secretes melatonin, a hormone that improves the quality and quantity of sleep. Therefore, reduced exposure to sunlight can have a detrimental effect on serotonin and melatonin, thus contributing to depressive symptoms.

## Postpartum Depression

A mild, usually transient form of depression may occur in as many as 70 percent of new mothers after they give birth. Women who experience postpartum depression feel a great sense of despair, cry easily for no apparent reason, and have difficulty sleeping. Some feel indifference toward their new infant, which can be quite distressing. Fortunately, postpartum depression dissipates within a few weeks for the majority of women; in some it persists, however, and turns into a major depression. Many of the factors discussed in this book may contribute to postpartum depression. These include deficiencies of certain important nutrients, such as iodine and omega-3 fatty acids, which preferentially go to the fetus during the pregnancy and to the baby during breast-feeding. Hormonal changes also play a role and can be addressed in various ways, to be discussed.

## Manic Depressive Illness, Bipolar Disorder, and Cyclothymic Disorder

Extreme mood swings, usually lasting weeks or months at a time, characterize manic depressive illness. During a manic phase, individuals may feel energized, euphoric, and overly self-confident; they may experience racing thoughts, be easily distracted, and find it difficult to sleep. Some people display reckless or inappropriate behavior, such as spending excessive amounts of money or engaging in promiscuous sex. Some patients may also become quite paranoid and suspicious of people and wind up with hallucinations (such as hearing voices that aren't there) or delusions (fixed false beliefs). When their mood swings the other way to depression, however, they are fatigued and extremely sad and withdraw from people and their environment.

Some individuals experience mood swings much more frequently than every few weeks or months. This condition is called bipolar disorder. Mood swings may occur as frequently as every few hours or even every few minutes. Various triggers may stimulate a manic episode in predisposed individuals, including environmental stresses, lack of sufficient rest, various stimulants, and many medications, including the ones used to treat depression.

Milder and less dramatic mood swings constitute a condition known as cyclothymia, which is a mild form of bipolar disorder. As I discuss the treatment of depression in this book, keep in mind the possibility that any given individual may have a tendency for mood swings and mania or bipolar disorder, especially if there is a family history of this condition. Consequently, it is important for the patient, his or her family, and the care-giving professional to be aware of this possibility and to deal with any swing toward mania or hypomania during the course of treatment by removing triggers, supplying calming nutrients and/or medications, and/or other calming methods discussed in this book.

## Anxiety Disorders

We will also consider anxiety disorders in our discussions because they often accompany depression, and because an orthomolecular/natural treatment approach is effective for these disorders as well. Generally, *anxiety* is defined as any unreasonable degree of uneasiness or apprehension about your past experiences, current situation, or the future. Here are the main types of anxiety disorders:

• **Generalized anxiety disorder.** Excessive, unrealistic worry that lasts six months or longer. Other symptoms may include muscle aches, insomnia, abdominal distress, excessive sweating, palpitations, irritability, and trembling.

• **Obsessive-compulsive disorder.** Characterized by persistent, recurring thoughts (obsessions) that reflect exaggerated fears or anxiety, such as excessive fear of germs. Obsessions may prompt individuals to perform rituals or routines (compulsions), like washing their hands dozens of times a day or hoarding food in an effort to relieve their anxiety.

• **Panic disorder.** Characterized by an overwhelming feeling of panic, which makes people feel as though they are going crazy or having a heart attack, yet there is no apparent reason for these feelings. Symptoms include chest pain or discomfort, sweating, trembling, heart palpitations, fear of dying, feelings of unreality, and tingling.

- **Post-traumatic stress disorder (PTSD).** This condition can follow exposure to a traumatic event, such as rape, witnessing a death, natural disaster, or the unexpected death of a loved one. Individuals with PTSD usually either relive the traumatic event in the form of nightmares or flashbacks; avoid places, people, or situations that are related to the trauma; or experience lingering physiological problems, such as irritability, poor concentration, or sleep difficulties.
- **Social anxiety disorder.** Characterized by extreme anxiety about being judged by others or behaving in an inappropriate or embarrassing manner. Physical symptoms include faintness, blushing, profuse sweating, and heart palpitations.
- **Phobias.** An intense fear reaction to a specific situation or object (say, flying, dogs, or heights) that is excessive and inappropriate to the situation, and that the affected individuals recognize as being irrational, even though they feel helpless to change it.

## SYMPTOM PROFILES

Symptom Profiles are tools you can use to help you identify the imbalances that may be contributing to or causing your depression. A Symptom Profile lists the typical signs and symptoms of imbalances of neurotransmitters, hormones, blood sugar, endorphins, fats, and essential fatty acids shown to be associated with depression and related mood disorders. You can use the Symptom Profiles when you move on to part 2 to help you choose, possibly with the help of a knowledgeable health-care professional, which natural approaches may work best for you.

As you look at the Symptom Profiles, you will see much overlap, indicating that there clearly is not a one-to-one correlation between a particular sign or symptom and a particular imbalance. Nevertheless, viewing the pattern of symptoms and signs can give clues to the type of imbalance. Also, there may be many combinations of imbalances, so each person must be evaluated as a unique individual.

## Serotonin Imbalance

Most of the serotonin in the body is manufactured by nerve cells that reside at the base of the brain in an area called the raphe nuclei, and it is made from the essential amino acid tryptophan, which is converted in the body to 5-hydroxytryptophan (5-HTP) and then to serotonin. These reactions in the body require certain nutrients to help them occur—vitamin $B_6$, vitamin C, and magnesium. Since tryptophan is capable of forming niacin (vitamin $B_3$) in the body, a deficiency of niacin will stimulate the body to convert tryptophan to niacin, resulting in relatively less tryptophan for conversion to serotonin. Conversely, supplying some niacin will inhibit the tryptophan pathway to niacin and promote serotonin production. Food sources of serotonin, which include meats, bananas, and pineapple, are considered less important because serotonin derived from food sources is destroyed in the body by enzymes in the gastrointestinal system before it gets to the brain.

#### CHARACTERISTICS OF SEROTONIN DEFICIENCY INCLUDE:

- Anxiety and a tendency to have panic attacks.
- Cravings for carbohydrates and sweets.
- Eating disorders.
- Fatigue.

- Impatience, irritability, and quickness to anger.
- Loss of sex drive.
- Low self-esteem and lack of confidence.
- Obsessive rumination or thoughts that can't be stopped.
- Angry, impulsive outbursts.
- Tendency toward alcohol or drug abuse.
- Various sleep problems.
- Dislike of cloudy days and tendency to be depressed during winter.
- Tendency to be shy or fearful.
- Inflexible behavior patterns that are hard to break.
- Phobias of all kinds, including fear of heights, snakes, or leaving the house.
- Tendency to be negative and pessimistic.
- Tendency to feel better when exercising.
- Premenstrual syndrome (PMS) in women.

## GABA Imbalance

Gamma aminobutyric acid (GABA) is an inhibitory neurotransmitter found in high concentrations in the brain, where it slows the transmission of signals among nerve cells. Because GABA slows things down, it can have a calming effect by reducing anxiety and stress, promoting sleep, and relaxing muscles. Some people refer to GABA as nature's Valium because of its calming effects.

### CHARACTERISTICS OF GABA DEFICIENCY INCLUDE:

- Frequent episodes of anxiety or nervousness.
- Feeling of exhaustion associated with stress.

- Panic attacks.
- Overreacting in stressful situations.
- Feelings of being overworked, pressured, or over-whelmed.
- Trouble relaxing and tense body.

## Dopamine Imbalance

We sometimes refer to dopamine as the pleasure neurotrans-mitter, because it transmits signals associated with pleasurable thoughts and experiences. It also plays a significant role in en-hancing mood and in cognitive functioning.

Positive events and situations, such as winning an award or getting a promotion, can raise dopamine levels in the brain. Un-fortunately, some mind-altering drugs (alcohol, cocaine, am-phetamines, marijuana, and nicotine, among others) can have the same effect. In fact, some drugs can raise your dopamine lev-els by up to 1,400 percent. Such a great increase is a burden to the brain, because it can't produce enough dopamine to meet the demand. Repeated use of these drugs often results in addiction, which causes damage to dopamine receptors and a decline in dopamine levels, followed by a depressed mood.

### CHARACTERISTICS OF DOPAMINE DEFICIENCY INCLUDE:

- Apathy and/or boredom.
- Sleeping a lot or other sleep disturbances.
- Irritability.
- Tendency to seek out and use stimulating substances, including alcohol, amphetamines, caffeine, cocaine, heroin, marijuana, nicotine, and sugar, to get self going.

- Have to push self to exercise.
- Trouble waking up in the morning.
- Tendency to put on weight too easily and have difficulty taking it off.

Elevated levels of dopamine in the brain can also cause mood-related challenges.

**CHARACTERISTICS OF ELEVATED LEVELS OF DOPAMINE INCLUDE:**

- Overly aggressive, impulsive, or irrational behavior.
- Tendency to take pleasurable activities, such as gambling, sex, eating, or exercise, to an addictive level.
- Sleep difficulties.

## Norepinephrine Imbalance

Most people associate norepinephrine (noradrenaline) with the fight-or-flight response: When a threatening situation occurs, norepinephrine is one of the main substances that surges through the body, increasing heart rate and breathing, and sending extra blood to the muscles. Yet this neurotransmitter is also associated with depression when there are low levels in the brain, which may be caused by excessive stress, insufficient protein in the diet, insufficient vitamin and mineral intake, and many other possible factors.

**CHARACTERISTICS OF NOREPINEPHRINE DEFICIENCY INCLUDE:**

- Foggy or sluggish thinking.
- Apathy.
- Lack of energy.

- Reduced sex drive.
- Anorexia and/or bulimia.

## Glutamine Deficiency

Glutamine is an amino acid and a critical component for optimal brain function. In particular, research indicates there is a connection between a glutamine deficiency and severe depression. This may be related to how it works in the brain: When it is carried to the brain through the bloodstream and crosses the blood–brain barrier, it is converted to glutamic acid (an excitatory neurotransmitter), which then may be converted to GABA (an inhibitory neurotransmitter), which is necessary for proper mental function.

#### CHARACTERISTICS OF GLUTAMINE DEFICIENCY INCLUDE:

- Tendency toward alcoholism.
- Cravings for sweets.
- Low sex drive.

## Endorphin Imbalance

Endorphins and enkephalins consist of a chain of amino acids often associated with pain relief; these chemicals, along with other similar ones, are the body's natural painkillers. Yet they also have a significant effect on mood and how the body responds to stress, which makes them important in our discussion.

Endorphins are released during exercise (they are what give runners and other endurance athletes their "runner's high"), as well as laughter and sex, and certain supplements and foods may increase their production.

**CHARACTERISTICS OF LOW LEVELS OF ENDORPHINS INCLUDE:**

- Anxiety.
- Phobias.
- Difficulty feeling pleasure.
- Tendency toward addictive behaviors (such as alcoholism or smoking) and obsessive-compulsive disorder.
- Inability to receive or give affection or love.

## Melatonin Imbalance

Light promotes the formation of melatonin but inhibits its release, while darkness promotes its release. The release of melatonin occurs primarily during the night and is associated with high-quality sleep, helping a person to remain asleep for an extended period without frequent awakenings. The pineal gland in the brain uses serotonin to make melatonin. Melatonin coordinates many functions in conjunction with the sleep–wake cycle. When melatonin levels are abnormally low or uncoordinated during sleep, mood disorders, sleep disorders, and behavioral changes are common occurrences. One study of major depression in children and adolescents, for example, found that melatonin levels were significantly lower in depressed patients with psychosis than in depressed patients without psychosis. Other research shows that unbalanced melatonin secretion is associated with depression in SAD.

**CHARACTERISTICS OF MELATONIN IMBALANCE OR
DEFICIENCY INCLUDE:**

- Seasonal affective disorder (SAD).
- Insomnia.

## Thyroid Dysfunction

Both reduced and elevated levels of thyroid hormones may be associated with depression. Low thyroid function, or hypothyroidism, is especially common among women and, unfortunately, often overlooked by physicians. Why? Because for various reasons, a person might have suboptimal thyroid functioning although blood tests appear to be normal. I will discuss reasons for this in a later chapter. Suffice it to say a person may have symptoms of an overactive or underactive thyroid and still have normal thyroid function tests. As will be emphasized in later chapters, previously unrecognized suboptimal iodine intake may be responsible for some thyroid-associated symptoms, and conventional medicine and public health policy may have contributed to this state of affairs.

**CHARACTERISTICS OF LOW THYROID FUNCTION INCLUDE:**

- Fatigue, lethargy, the need to sleep more than eight hours, poor energy level.
- Tendency to gain weight or an inability to lose weight despite a sensible diet.
- Mental fog, difficulty with concentration and/or memory.
- Tendency to feel cold, especially the hands and feet.
- Low blood pressure and/or slow heart rate.
- Low body temperature.
- Tendency to retain fluids; swollen face, feet, and eyelids are some indications.
- Headaches and/or migraines.
- Feeling of a lump in the throat.
- Reduced sex drive.

- Menstrual problems, including excessive bleeding, irregular periods, severe cramping, and severe PMS symptoms.
- Hoarseness.
- High cholesterol levels.
- Brittle nails.
- Coarse, dry hair.

### CHARACTERISTICS OF ELEVATED THYROID HORMONE LEVELS INCLUDE:

- Fatigue.
- Anxiety, nervousness, and/or irritability.
- Increased perspiration.
- Weight loss.
- Diarrhea.
- Protruding eyeballs.
- Tremors of the hands.
- Sensitivity to heat.
- Rapid heartbeat.

## Stress Hormone Imbalance

The body responds to and deals with stress—be it physical, chemical (drugs, toxins), or emotional—in many ways. One of the main responses is the secretion of specific hormones produced by the structures that play a significant role in handling stress: the hypothalamus, the pituitary, and the adrenals. When the body is under stress, these three work together as a unit called the HPA (hypothalamic-pituitary-adrenal axis), which I explain briefly here but in more detail in chapter 9.

For example, when the hypothalamus, which lies deep

within the brain, receives stress signals from the body, it produces corticotropin-releasing hormone (or factor, sometimes abbreviated CRF). This hormone stimulates the pituitary (which lies at the base of the brain) to produce another hormone, adrenocorticotropic hormone (ACTH), which races through the bloodstream to the adrenals. The adrenals are then stimulated to secrete corticosteroids (cortisol, cortisone, and corticosterone) from their outer layers (the adrenal cortex). The adrenal gland also has an inner portion called the adrenal medulla that secretes epinephrine and norepinephrine (the fight-or-flight hormones) under conditions of acute stress.

The body strives to maintain a balance among these hormones. Thus, if cortisol levels in the blood are too high, the pituitary reacts by producing less adrenocorticotropic hormone. But when the body is under frequent or continuous stress, the delicate hormone balance can be disrupted, causing or exacerbating existing depression.

### CHARACTERISTICS OF IMBALANCE IN THE STRESS HORMONE SYSTEM INCLUDE:

- Fatigue.
- Anxiety.
- Headache.
- Muscle pain.
- Poor wound healing.
- Overall weakness.
- Problems with memory.
- Weight gain.

## Blood Sugar Imbalance

For optimal functioning, your brain relies on sugar (glucose), as do your other organs and muscles. Naturally, it's not as simple as just making sure your brain has an adequate amount of sugar; there are many other elements involved in breaking down sugar to produce the basic energy molecular compound known as adenosine triphosphate (ATP), which is utilized by the brain. Yet if your blood sugar is out of balance, it throws a monkey wrench into the process of supplying ATP to the brain, and may result in depression and other impaired mental functioning.

### CHARACTERISTICS OF BLOOD SUGAR IMBALANCE INCLUDE:

- Nervousness.
- Weakness.
- Dizziness, faintness.
- Drowsiness.
- Mental confusion and problems with concentration.
- Cravings for sweets or alcohol.
- Heart palpitations.
- Problems with coordination.
- Frequent yawning and sighing.
- Anxiety.
- Irritability.
- Insomnia.
- Crying spells.
- Leg cramps.

## Fat/Fatty Acid Imbalance

Optimal health demands that your body has sufficient levels of beneficial fats while avoiding harmful fats as much as possible. Thus, you want to optimize and balance your essential fatty acids and minimize your exposure to toxic fats, such as transfatty acids.

#### CHARACTERISTICS OF FATTY ACID IMBALANCE INCLUDE:

- Fatigue.
- Dry skin.
- Lack of appetite.
- Constipation.
- Vision difficulties.
- Overall weakness.
- Headache.
- Minor skin problems.
- Brittle fingernails.
- Hair loss.
- Weakened immune system (characterized by frequent colds, flu, infections).
- Nervousness.
- Inflammatory conditions, such as arthritis.
- Tingling in the arms and legs.
- Slow metabolism.

## Other Indicators

As discussed in chapters 1 and 2, poor diet, exposure to toxins, underlying medical conditions, and use of various prescription, over-the-counter, and illicit drugs can contribute to depression. Your health-care professionals should identify these indicators during your initial evaluations and testing procedures. To help this process, be sure to provide complete, accurate information regarding your personal medical history, family medical history, dietary habits, and drug use.

## NEUROTRANSMITTER TESTING

Neurotransmitter testing is a new, exciting, and, I believe, critically important tool in the treatment of depression and other conditions that are related to neurotransmitter imbalances. One reason why this testing is so exciting is that although the use of amino acid therapy has been around since the 1970s, until recently there has been no reliable way to analyze neurotransmitter levels, nor any established reference ranges for the neurotransmitters that physicians could use to help them make treatment decisions.

That has changed somewhat, because measuring neurotransmitters in the urine can be helpful in figuring out what is happening to neurotransmitters in the brain, though the correlation is clearly not one-to-one. Interpretation in conjunction with the symptoms of the patient and the clinical and laboratory changes over time in response to treatment are necessary. Neurotransmitter testing, interpretation, and therapy are still relatively new and thus rapidly changing, but we now have reliable ways to evaluate neurotransmitter levels in the urine.

Neurotransmitter testing and some other diagnostic tests, mentioned on pages 69 to 74, are helpful if you want to find the most effective approach to treating your depression. This includes use of the Symptom Profile lists, which can help you identify which factors may be the cause of your depression.

Symptoms alone do not accurately identify an imbalance: Two people may report feeling depressed, anxious, and unable to concentrate, yet have very different imbalances contributing to their symptoms. That's why neurotransmitter testing is a much-needed addition to the diagnostic process in the treatment of depression.

## How Testing Is Done

The testing process is very simple. Patients are given a specimen collection kit, which instructs them to collect a single urine sample around 11 AM after the first voided urine of the day. They mail the specimen directly to the laboratory, where it is analyzed, and the results are sent to the patient's physician.

These baseline results are compared against a reference optimal range, which was established by measuring neurotransmitter levels in people who were feeling and functioning well. The information from this test is used along with results from other tests to choose a course of amino acid therapy. (We also begin other treatments, but here I am referring to amino acid therapy only.) After about two months of treatment, the neurotransmitter test is repeated to determine if the chosen amino acid therapy is making a difference in neurotransmitter levels. The results of the test in conjunction with changes in symptoms are then used to determine if any changes need to be made in the therapeutic program. Your health-care practitioner may retest again in several months depending on your progress.

## Sample Neurotransmitter Test Results

### Average of Sample Collected

|  | NT Evaluated Baseline | Retest 1 | Retest 2 | Optimal Range |
|---|---|---|---|---|
| Epinephrine | 3.1 | 3.9 | 5.4 | 8–12 |
| Norepinephrine | 24.2 | 56.1 | 51.1 | 30–55 |
| Dopamine | 95.7 | 345.7 | 199.5 | 125–175 |
| Serotonin | 101.5 | 789.2 | 245.4 | 175–225 |
| GABA | 4.9 | 4.1 | 4.0 | 2–4 |

The table above shows the neurotransmitter test results of one patient, Patricia, who was treated with amino acid therapy for depression and fatigue. As you can see, all of her neurotransmitter levels were out of optimal range when she first came to be tested. After four months (her first retest was at two months, her second at four months) of amino acid therapy and dietary changes, all of her neurotransmitter levels had changed significantly and moved toward optimal levels. More important, she was feeling 100 percent better and, for the first time in five years, had the energy and motivation to initiate a career change.

### DIAGNOSTIC TESTS

In addition to neurotransmitter testing, there are dozens of other tests we can use to identify biochemical changes and imbalances, as well as other contributory factors that may be associated with depressive mood. The following list is a summary of many of the tests we use at the Schachter Center, which you may encounter during your evaluation process. "Sample" refers to the type of sample needed to conduct the study.

• **Amino acid test.** Assesses amino acid levels, which may show evidence of low protein intake, specific amino acid deficiencies or excesses, inborn errors of metabolism, and evidence of nutrient deficiencies. Sample: serum or urine.

• **Complete blood count (CBC).** Measures red blood cells, white blood cells, and platelets, along with associated indices. Screens for a variety of disorders, including anemia, evidence of infection, certain nutritional deficiencies, and exposure to toxins. Sample: whole blood.

• **Comprehensive metabolic profile.** A routine series of tests performed to analyze components of the blood, including glucose, liver enzymes, bilirubin, calcium, phosphorus, sodium, potassium, chloride, kidney function (BUN and creatinine), globulin, and albumin. Screens for a variety of body functions and possible diseases. Sample: serum.

• **Cortisol.** This major stress hormone from the adrenal cortex is probably best evaluated by taking four or five samples during the day because of daytime variation. Sample: saliva.

• **C-reactive protein.** Helps identify the presence of inflammation. Sample: serum.

• **DHEA sulfate.** Determines if DHEA concentrations are normal and helps evaluate adrenal function. Sample: serum; DHEA can be measured in saliva.

• **Digestive stool analysis (comprehensive).** Supplies information about gastrointestinal function and possible disorders. From a stool sample, information can be obtained about deficiencies in stomach acid, digestive enzymes, malabsorption, pathological bacteria, and fungi. Sample: fecal material.

- **Dimercaptosuccinic acid (DMSA) challenge for toxic metals.** DMSA is a chelating agent that binds to toxic heavy metals, such as lead, cadmium, and mercury, and helps to remove them from the body through the urine. A DMSA capsule is given and the patient collects urine usually for six hours; a laboratory measures toxic heavy metals to determine if the patient may be suffering from an increase in heavy metals. Sample: urine.

- **Erythrocyte sedimentation rate (ESR).** Used to detect and monitor the activity of inflammation to help determine if inflammation is playing a role in the patient's condition. Sample: whole blood.

- **Ferritin.** This protein binds iron in the body and correlates with the overall iron content of the body. Low levels indicate an iron deficiency; high levels, an overload. Each of these conditions needs to be corrected. Sample: serum.

- **Fibrinogen.** This protein plays a role in the blood-clotting process in the body. When it is too high, the blood will tend to clot too easily and thereby increase the risk of a stroke or heart attack. Diet and supplements can help to correct this condition. Sample: whole blood.

- **Folic acid.** A very important B vitamin that is frequently low in depressed patients. In more advanced cases, it may contribute to anemia or nerve damage. Sample: serum.

- *Helicobacter pylori* **antibodies.** The presence of positive antibodies to *H. pylori* often indicates an *H. pylori* infection, which may contribute to gastrointestinal complaints as well as anxiety and depression in some cases. Sample: serum.

- **Homocysteine.** This amino acid derivative is, when elevated, a significant risk factor for heart attack, stroke, and Alzheimer's disease. It may also be high in some depressed patients and indicate a deficiency in one or more of several nutrients, including folic acid, vitamin $B_6$, vitamin $B_{12}$, or a methyl donor such as trimethylglycine. It is one of the markers that relates to methylation (to be discussed at the beginning of part 2 in this book). Sample: serum.

• **Iodine loading test.** A patient empties his bladder and then ingests 50 mg of iodine/iodide as liquid drops or tablets or capsules. Urine is collected for twenty-four hours and a sample, along with a note as to the total amount of urine collected over this period, is sent to a laboratory. The total amount of iodine excreted is then calculated. According to some investigators, an iodine-sufficient person should excrete about 90 percent or 45 of the 50 mg. This test is in the process of being validated. Sample: urine.

• **Lipid profile.** Provides levels of total cholesterol, high-density lipoprotein (HDL) cholesterol, low-density lipoprotein (LDL) cholesterol, and triglycerides. High LDL and triglycerides and low HDL indicate an increased risk for cardiovascular events. Sample: serum.

• **Lipoprotein (a) test.** This is another risk factor for heart disease, stroke, and death. When test results are high, the condition can be treated with certain amino acids and vitamin C. Sample: serum.

• **Methylmalonic acid test.** Elevated levels of this chemical in the blood or urine indicate a deficiency of vitamin $B_{12}$ and/or certain genetic disorders. Sample: serum or urine.

• **Organic acid test.** Evaluates numerous organic acid compounds, focusing on yeast and bacteria by-products absorbed from the gastrointestinal tract and excreted in the urine; also provides evidence for nutritional and antioxidant deficiencies, amino acid abnormalities, fatty acid abnormalities, and others. Sample: urine.

• **Red blood cell fatty acids.** Reflects the status of fatty acids in the body, including essential fatty acids and toxic fatty acids, such as trans-fatty acids. Sample: packed red blood cells.

• **Red blood cell minerals test.** Screens for levels of minerals (nutritional and toxic) inside red blood cells, which may reflect deficiencies or toxicity of minerals. Sample: blood.

• **Thyroid antibodies.** Positive antibodies to the thyroid suggest chronic inflammation of the thyroid (Hashimoto's disease or thyroiditis) and indicates a thyroid problem even when thyroid function tests are normal. Sample: serum.

• **Thyroid profile.** Determines T3, T4, and thyroid-stimulating hormone (TSH) to help identify thyroid disorders. Sample: serum.

• **Urinalysis.** Screens for metabolic and kidney disorders. Sample: urine.

• **Vitamin B$_{12}$.** Low vitamin B$_{12}$ often results in fatigue and depression. More advanced B$_{12}$ deficiency may lead to anemia and nerve damage, just like folic acid. This test and the one for folic acid are usually done together. Sample: serum.

• **Vitamin levels.** Many other vitamin levels may be measured, such as vitamin A, various members of the B complex, vitamin C, vitamin D, and other nutrients to check for deficiencies. Sample: serum or frozen serum.

## FINDING PROFESSIONAL HELP

By now, you're aware that depression is a complex condition, requiring a multifaceted approach that addresses your specific circumstances. The one-size-fits-all medication dispensed by a physician who has spent very little time with you and who does not have a detailed profile of your biochemical makeup is often not the answer. You need a professional who will work with you to identify any imbalances, institute orthomolecular and natural methods to correct them, help you modify your lifestyle to incorporate treatment methods, and introduce drugs only if and when necessary. Sometimes you may need a team of professionals, such as a psychiatrist and a nutritionist, because one person may not have all of the skills necessary to administer a comprehensive approach.

So what types of professionals might be helpful? Medical doctors (MDs) and/or osteopathic physicians (DOs) who have similar conventional training and who have an interest and some training in nutritional, complementary, integrative, or orthomolecular medicine would be a good place to start. If they have also been trained in conventional psychiatry, this would be another advantage.

Naturopathic physicians who have gone through a licensed and/or certified four-year naturopathic medical school might also be considered. Unfortunately, only about a dozen states license this group of professionals. These physicians have probably been trained in many of the modalities discussed in this book, but are generally not able to prescribe psychotropic medications. If medications are needed, an MD, DO, or nurse practitioner would have to be utilized in addition to the naturopathic physician. The American Association of Naturopathic Physicians (AANP; see appendix) has a database of all naturopathic physicians who have graduated from recognized four-year naturopathic schools. Other naturopaths may also be helpful.

Psychiatrists are the best trained in prescribing psychotropic medication, but many of them tend to deny the value of any other treatment approach and may have difficulty working with a patient who is utilizing some of the treatment modalities discussed in this book.

Certified nutritionists and/or chiropractors trained in nutritional medicine may offer some help. Classical homeopaths, discussed in chapter 11, offer another effective approach for some people. Several homeopathic organizations are listed in the appendix.

I supply the names and websites of some organizations in the appendix that might help you to find a professional who approaches depression in the way discussed in this book.

Does finding professional help sound like a tall order? Well, it can be, especially in certain areas of the country, but it certainly is doable. You might start with your local telephone directory under "Physicians" and look for the subheadings "Orthomolecular," "Complementary," "Integrative," and/or "Holistic." You can also contact various organizations to help you find such professionals in your area. These include the American Academy of Environmental Medicine (AAEM), the American College for Advancement in Medicine (ACAM), and the Institute for Functional Medicine (IFN), among others. They maintain lists of physicians, which may include their interest and specialties. Contact information for these organizations is in the appendix. However, it is important to contact the specific practitioner's office and determine what diagnostic and treatment modalities he or she uses, as well as his or her training and qualifications, especially in treating depression. You may need to determine if the professional is willing to work with other professionals in your care if he or she doesn't have all of the skills you would like to utilize in your treatment.

Once you've identified a practitioner who seems to match the needs outlined above, you should learn as much as you can about him or her:

- Do you know anyone who is being treated by the doctor? If possible, talking with current patients could help you make your decision.
- Does he or she give lectures or talks around town? If yes, make a point of attending them. Such events often include a question-and-answer session, which will give you an opportunity to learn more about the practitioner and to ask questions.
- Has he or she published any articles in professional or consumer journals or magazines? You can look for such information on the Internet by either conducting a general search on a major search engine, or by going to the National Library of Medicine website: www.nlm.nih.gov.

## Choosing a Doctor

Here are a few other questions you should ask before you make your final decision.

- Where did the doctor attend medical or osteopathic school, and what type of postgraduate training did he or she have? You can verify your doctor's training and certification status through the American Medical Association's Physician Select, a free service that can be accessed at www.ama-assn.org/aps/amahg.htm.
- How many years has the doctor been practicing?

- Does the doctor have a solo or group practice? If it is a group practice, who will see you if your doctor is not available? You should know the background of each of the other practitioners in the practice with whom you may interact.

- Has the doctor ever been convicted of fraud, been reprimanded by the state disciplinary board, or had any action taken against him or her? Each state has a medical board that keeps a record of disciplined doctors. You can contact your state medical board directly, or you can visit a central location on the Internet that has links to the states' medical boards: the Public Citizen Research Group, a free service that can be accessed at www.citizen .org/hrg/publications/1506.htm. One caution: Some state licensing boards are biased against alternative approaches that deviate from conventional medical or psychiatric protocols. As a result, some excellent alternative or orthomolecular physicians have been disciplined by their medical board simply for practicing in a manner that differed from that of most conventional physicians. Consequently, a physician should not automatically be eliminated from consideration simply because he or she has been disciplined. Learn the reasons for the disciplinary action.

- Is the doctor available on weekends or at night for emergency phone calls?

- Are the doctor's office location and hours convenient for you?

## THE DIAGNOSTIC PROCESS

Every health-care practitioner has his or her own approach and methods for gathering information to begin the diagnostic process. I will share with you the assessment process that we use at the Schachter Center. The point I want to emphasize here is this: *An individual who is depressed can have many different kinds of imbalances, so it is crucial to identify each person's unique biochemical identity as well as other unique qualities.* Once this identity is established, an educated treatment decision can be made.

Our initial diagnostic visit may take ninety minutes or longer and is often conducted by a certified physician's assistant (PA-C). During this visit, the PA-C will take a comprehensive personal and family medical history, develop Symptom Profiles with the patient, conduct a physical examination, and order laboratory tests, such as a complete blood count, urinalysis, a comprehensive metabolic panel, thyroid panel, cholesterol lipid panel, homocysteine, C-reactive protein, red blood cell minerals test, and any others that are indicated by the information provided and any signs and symptoms noted.

At this time, neurotransmitter testing may also be ordered for the patient to do at home. Information from this important testing procedure helps health-care practitioners like me to not only choose the most appropriate treatment options, but also monitor a patient's progress and make informed changes to treatment along the way.

Based on the initial information obtained from the first visit, a preliminary plan is outlined for the patient. This program is modified during subsequent visits after the test results are returned and the patient reports on the effects of the initial program.

A visit with a nutritionist may also be part of the initial evaluation. Very few people eat a healthful diet, so a nutritionist can evaluate your diet and make some specific recommendations, even before test results have been returned. At the Schachter Center, I have a "Foods to Avoid" list, which I share in chapter 7, and which I give to all patients on their initial visit. Once a patient's test results come back, we can adjust the dietary recommendations as needed.

At the initial evaluation, arrangements are sometimes made for a program of injectable nutrients, such as vitamin C, calcium and magnesium, and B vitamins, as well as psychotherapy, classical homeopathy, or acupuncture within or outside the Schachter Center, depending upon the needs of the patient.

In most cases, I see the patient within a few weeks after laboratory tests are back. This is a time when I review test results with the patient, recommend additional tests if indicated, and implement a more precise treatment plan that may include targeted amino acid therapy, hormone therapy, nutritional guidelines, and mind–body work. The patient is evaluated again for other referrals, such as psychotherapy, classical homeopathy, or acupuncture, if this has not yet been implemented.

Although the procedure described above is most often followed at my center, in some cases it is more appropriate for me to consult with the patient before a meeting with the physician's assistant; I will do this if the patient requests it or if I think it is more appropriate, as long as my schedule allows. At this visit, I assess the patient's needs and may recommend a full workup that begins with an evaluation by the PA-C and continues with the procedure described above.

## THE BOTTOM LINE

It is important for you to participate fully in your evaluation and treatment. Some people will be able to learn enough from this book to set the healing process in motion and achieve satisfactory results. Others will do better to seek the help of a qualified professional who knows how to identify and correct the various imbalances and other factors causing depression. In most cases, when possible, it is best to find a practitioner who is knowledgeable to aid you in your quest for health. In this chapter, I provided you with an arsenal of tools to help identify the factors contributing to and causing your depressive mood and associated symptoms. Now it's time to begin using those tools to initiate the healing process.

# Part 2

————— ❦ —————

# HOW TO PREVENT AND TREAT DEPRESSION COMPREHENSIVELY

In the quest to uncover the causes of depression and other mood disorders, we often need to seek answers at the cellular and molecular level. Although the biochemical processes that occur at this level are complex, I believe it's important for you to understand some of the basic concepts, because they have a significant impact on how I treat depression, and specifically on what supplements I recommend. The two important interrelated mechanisms that I will discuss are methylation and transsulfuration, both of which are essential to life and relate to mood regulation. I suggest you use the figure on page 84, which diagrams these processes, as you follow along in the text.

You could skip the next few pages and still obtain enough information and tools from this book to put you on the road to recovery. However, *the processes I am about to describe play an integral part in the most important treatments discussed in this book,* and I believe a fuller understanding of them will only enhance your recovery. Therefore I encourage you to bear with me as I describe, as simply as possible, the critical role these two processes play in depression and mood disorders. I also encourage you to refer back to this section as needed as you read the chapters that follow.

## Methionine Metabolism
## Showing Methylation and Transsulfuration

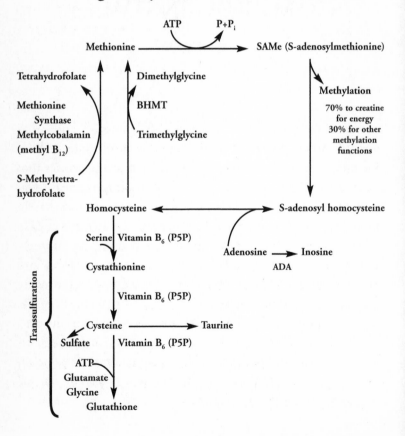

## METHYLATION

Methylation is a process by which a methyl group (one carbon atom attached to three hydrogen atoms) is transferred from one molecule to another. These transfers occur millions of times every minute of your life and are essential for detoxifying poisons from the body, manufacturing hormones, changing one neurotransmitter to another, synchronizing neural networks to allow for smooth functioning of the nervous system in terms of cognition and mood regulation, making DNA and RNA, and other functions. Methylation allows different areas of the brain to work in harmony, which helps people to pay attention and integrate their emotions with perception and thinking, all of which has an important effect on mood regulation.

Molecules that possess methyl groups for transfer are called *methyl donors*, and include methionine, SAMe, dimethyl-glycine, trimethylglycine, and choline. Of these, the amino acid methionine is the most abundant methyl donor, but most methyl transfers throughout the body are accomplished by S-adenosylmethione (SAMe), which is formed when methionine is activated by adenosine triphosphate (ATP; see page 86).

To facilitate the methylation process, methyl donors get help from *methylating factors*. Zinc, vitamin $B_{12}$, and folic acid are methylating factors, and their job is either to help enzymes that detach methyl groups from methyl donors and reattach them to other molecules, or to help in the recycling of methyl groups. Certain enzymes involved in this process are easily poisoned by mercury and other toxic minerals. Therefore, methylation can be inhibited by these toxins, which can lead to mood changes and other problems.

Let's look at methylation using methionine as our starting point. Methionine comes from dietary protein and contains both sulfur (involved in transsulfuration) and a methyl group (involved in methylation). Methionine reacts with magnesium and ATP, the major supplier of energy for most of the energy-consuming activities of cells. The result of this reaction is the formation of SAMe, a substance that contributes to the synthesis of melatonin (from serotonin), epinephrine, and choline, among others, and which is an important methyl donor for neurotransmitters. (See chapters 4 and 6 for more on SAMe.)

About 70 percent of the SAMe that is formed (and not recycled) donates its methyl group to creatine to form creatine phosphate, which is used for energy reactions throughout the body, including the brain. Thus, problems with methylation can result in fatigue, brain fog, and many other symptoms associated with depression. The other 30 percent is used for other methylation reactions in the body. The picture thus far is: methionine + ATP/magnesium = SAMe, which can give off its methyl group to a variety of substances.

When SAMe donates a methyl group, it converts into another substance called homocysteine, an amino acid in the blood that, at elevated levels, can cause narrowing and hardening of the arteries, which in turn can result in heart attack or stroke.

So, SAMe – methyl group = homocysteine. Homocysteine can then take one of two pathways, both of which are important for good mental and overall health.

First, homocysteine can be converted back to methionine for conversion to SAMe as described above. To recycle homocysteine to methionine requires that folic acid transfer a methyl group to vitamin $B_{12}$ to form methylcobalamin, or methyl $B_{12}$. Methyl $B_{12}$, with the help of folic acid, transfers this methyl group to homocysteine to re-form methionine. In many cases, injections of methyl $B_{12}$ can help support methylation and improve the symptoms associated with depression.

The second path homocysteine may take is transsulfuration, which involves the movement of sulfur.

## TRANSSULFURATION

In transsulfuration, homocysteine is converted to the amino acid cysteine, which can then be converted to glutathione, sulfate, or taurine. Sulfur is important in many compounds that involve detoxification and neutralization of free radicals. When this pathway is taken, the methionine is lost and must be restored through diet. The conversion of homocysteine to cysteine (a nonessential amino acid containing sulfur) takes place in two steps, both of which require vitamin $B_6$ and magnesium.

You don't need to understand all aspects of transsulfuration except to know that the cysteine that results from it is a precursor of reduced glutathione (GSH—a term that refers to the metabolically active form of glutathione), a substance that transports mercury and other toxins out of cells (see chapter 8). To get glutathione, cysteine is joined by glutamate (a neurotransmitter), ATP, and glycine (an amino acid), as follows: cysteine + glutamate + ATP + glycine = glutathione.

Glutathione is the most important intracellular antioxidant and helps to maintain a favorable environment for the body's chemistry. Various toxins, free radicals, and toxic minerals such as mercury and lead use up reduced glutathione.

Depletion of reduced glutathione in the body is a major factor in depression and many other disease conditions.

Other important compounds are made from cysteine via this pathway. One is taurine, which helps inhibitory neurotransmitters; another is sulfate, which is important in the liver for detoxifying substances in preparation for them to be removed from the body.

## WHY METHYLATION AND TRANSSULFURATION MATTER

It is important to understand the competition that occurs between the homocysteine pathways: Homocysteine can either convert back to methionine, or it can convert to cysteine and glutathione. So, for example, if the body is under a lot of toxic stress that requires antioxidant activity, more cysteine and glutathione will be formed, which will result in less SAMe being available for methylation. One consequence of this SAMe insufficiency will be less formation of creatine, which will result in reduced available energy for the body and particularly the brain. This can affect mood.

Methylation can be effective only if methionine, the necessary enzymes, and appropriate cofactors are available. If your diet is deficient in methionine, both methylation and transsulfuration will be reduced, resulting in problems. A deficiency of folic acid and/or vitamin $B_{12}$, for example, can result in an impaired ability to regenerate methionine and thus cause elevated homocysteine levels, a state that is associated with depression, heart disease, fatigue, low thyroid function, cognitive decline, and irritable bowel syndrome. A deficiency of vitamin $B_6$ can reduce the ability to form cysteine and glutathione from homocysteine and also cause an elevation of homocysteine.

I strongly recommend having your homocysteine levels checked. Generally, levels below 9 mmol/L (millimoles per liter) are considered normal, though there is some evidence to indicate that going to levels of 6 or 7 is optimal. Thus, for better mental health as well as heart health, it's important to improve methylation. Fortunately, this can be done with the appropriate foods, detoxification, and supplements.

Sources of methionine include fish, cheese, eggs, meat, poultry, and sunflower seeds, with lesser amounts in fruits, vegetables, and fermented foods. People who don't get enough methionine can take a supplement or another methyl donor, trimethylglycine or SAMe, to enhance methylation. To ensure that you get enough vitamin $B_6$, $B_{12}$, and folic acid, eat foods rich in these nutrients and take supplements. I also recommend you avoid refined sugars and limit fats; excesses of these elements deplete folic acid and vitamin $B_6$.

I've only scratched the surface of methylation and transsulfuration, but the take-home message is that a glitch in these processes due to a deficiency of any of the components can have a critical impact on mood. That's why it's essential to tackle depression from all fronts—amino acid therapy, proper diet, supplementation, hormone therapy, essential fatty acids, and lifestyle modifications—all of which are discussed in the chapters that follow. You'll also be reading more about the many components of methylation and transsulfuration throughout this book.

## Chapter 4

# Up with Amino Acids

When it comes to balancing the brain's levels of neurotransmitters and the body's hormone and endorphin levels, the star players are amino acids, which I believe are the frontline treatment for depression. Again and again I have seen how identifying neurotransmitter imbalances and then adding just the right amino acids through food and/or supplementation to help rebalance those levels has brought positive mood changes, occasionally in as brief a time as a day or two. These amazing molecules can do what antidepressant drugs cannot—they allow the body to increase the levels of neurotransmitters in the brain, naturally and safely. Unlike most neurotransmitters, amino acids can cross the blood–brain barrier and thus function as *precursors*—substances that precede and are the source of another substance—and facilitate production of specific neurotransmitters, as well as hormones and endorphins (see chapter 1), that have an impact on mood.

Although I've talked about amino acids in previous chapters and specifically introduced methionine and the processes of methylation and transsulfuration in the introduction to part 2, here is where you will learn what you need to know about these powerhouses against depression. You'll discover which neurotransmitters each amino acid influences, and—best of all—use the information from your checklists to identify which amino acids are most likely to improve your mood. You'll also discover which types of symptoms each amino acid can treat effectively, how to incorporate amino acids into your lifestyle, and how amino acid therapy can be used along with drugs, when the latter are necessary, to optimize the effect of both methods of treatment.

## WHAT ARE AMINO ACIDS?

Amino acids are relatively small nitrogen-containing molecules used by the body to manufacture moderate-size chains of amino acids called *peptides* and larger chains called *proteins*. Conversely, you need to consume protein in your diet so that your body can break it down into moderate-size chains of amino acids called *polypeptides* with the help of digestive enzymes produced by the body. The polypeptides are then further broken down by digestive enzymes into amino acids so they can be absorbed into the body through the small intestine. Like essential vitamins that generally cannot be made by the body, but must be ingested in the diet or via supplements, the *essential amino acids* can't be made by the body. Others can be made in the body from the essential amino acids; these are the *nonessential amino acids.*

Some of those amino acids—less than half of the twenty-two that have been identified in humans—play varying roles in maintaining a balanced mood and banishing depression. The amino acids with the most influence on mood, sleep patterns, sexual arousal, and other functions include tryptophan, 5-HTP (5-hydroxytryptophan), GABA (gamma aminobutyric acid), glutamine, phenylalanine, and tyrosine; those with a lesser but still noteworthy role include taurine, methionine, cysteine, theanine, histidine, and a metabolite of methionine called S-adenosylmethionine or SAMe.

I and other practitioners who use amino acid therapy to treat depression call upon what we know about how each of these amino acids function in the body to determine which ones we will prescribe for any given patient, based on his or her symptoms, as well as laboratory tests. On that note, there are four important points I want to make here:

- Because depression and other related symptoms are often the result of an imbalance in more than one neurotransmitter, more than one amino acid usually must be prescribed.
- Neurotransmitters can be classified as inhibitory or excitatory. Inhibitory neurotransmitters are involved with relaxation, calming down the system, and helping you focus. If inhibition is overactive, the result is likely to be lethargy and poor motivation. Excitatory neurotransmitters are generally involved in motivation, accomplishing tasks, active thinking, and similar functions. When excitatory neurotransmitters are overactive, anxiety, agitation, and even violence may result.
- Amino acids are generally prescribed in three phases. During the first phase, those that balance the inhibitory system are selected. The goal is to reduce depression and anxiety and regulate the stimulatory effects of excitatory neurotransmitters—in effect, bringing the inhibitory

system into balance. During the second phase, amino acids that affect the excitatory neurotransmitters are prescribed, which helps bring the excitatory system into balance. Your physician will need to retest your neurotransmitter levels occasionally and make amino acid dose adjustments over time until your neurotransmitters are in a range that is healthy for you and your symptoms have resolved. During the third phase, the goal is to adjust the amino acid doses to maintain neurotransmitter levels in the optimal range.

• Unlike many conventional psychiatrists, *I believe that in some cases, amino acid therapy and drug therapy can complement each other.* The amino acids increase the levels of available neurotransmitters, and the drugs work to ensure that the neurotransmitters are where they need to be to relieve depression. For a further discussion of the use of antidepressants and other drugs used to treat mood disorders, see chapter 12.

In discussions of amino acid therapy, you may see the prefix *L-, D-,* or *DL-* as part of the name of the amino acid. These prefixes refer to how the atoms of the amino acid molecules are arranged in space—as mirror images of each other. There are really two forms, L- and D-, because DL- is simply a mixture of the two. Most of the amino acids in humans and most amino acid supplements are in the L- form, although there are a few exceptions. The L- forms are much more commonly used than the other two forms and therefore, unless otherwise stated, I am referring to the L- form of amino acids in this chapter and the rest of the book.

If you have chosen the Symptom Profiles presented in

chapter 3 that most typify your depression, you're ready to look at the following amino acids to see which can help you on the road to becoming depression-free. First, however, let's look at what makes amino acid therapy so special and why you and your psychiatrist or primary health-care practitioner need to talk about it.

## AMINO ACID THERAPY

Experts have known for decades that amino acids play a significant role in mood disorders and have conducted many studies to uncover ways to use them most effectively. In the late 1950s, for example, researchers discovered that 5-HTP can lead to increased serotonin levels; in the early 1970s, tryptophan was used in studies of depression. As amino acid therapy began to gain some attention in the 1980s, numerous pharmaceutical companies introduced a new class of antidepressants to the market—selective serotonin reuptake inhibitors, or SSRIs. At around the same time, a contaminated batch of tryptophan from Japan caused a serious potentially fatal disease (eosinophilia-myalgia syndrome), and the Food and Drug Administration removed tryptophan from the market. Contamination may have been caused by a change in production procedure, but this has never been fully clarified. The FDA's response was appropriate, since at the time it wasn't clear whether a contaminant or the tryptophan itself caused this severe reaction. With the introduction of SSRIs and with tryptophan no longer being available, amino acid therapy took a backseat as millions of prescriptions were written for these new drugs. Unfortunately, these drugs didn't—and still don't—address the issue of depletion of neurotransmitters, which may be the source of depression. Frequently, prescription drugs provide only a temporary fix or do not help at all, while causing side effects. (For more on prescription drugs for depression, see chapter 12.)

Today, advances in research of neurotransmitters and amino acid therapy for depression and associated mood disorders have made it possible to not only estimate neurotransmitter levels in the brain but also target the use of amino acids to modify the levels of specific neurotransmitters. Amino acid therapy has left the lab and entered the real world, and practitioners like me can offer it to our patients with confidence. At present, changes are occurring rapidly in the field of amino acid therapy, so I think we can expect modifications in treatment approaches and improved therapeutic results in the near future.

As mentioned above, neurotransmitters can generally be classified as primarily either inhibitory or excitatory. The major inhibitory neurotransmitter is GABA; the major excitatory neurotransmitter is glutamate. Neurotransmitters and/or substances that enhance the inhibitory neurotransmitters include serotonin, theanine, taurine, and glycine. Those that enhance the excitatory system include dopamine, norepinephrine, epinephrine, and phenylethylamine (PEA).

## 5-HTP (5-HYDROXYTRYPTOPHAN)

If you are deficient in serotonin, a quick, safe way for your body to produce the serotonin it needs is to take a supplement containing 5-hydroxytryptophan or 5-HTP. This amino acid is converted directly into the neurotransmitter serotonin, as shown here:

### 5-HTP → Serotonin

Of interest is that 5-HTP is not generally found in food, but is made in the body from the essential amino acid tryptophan. If you don't have a sufficient supply of tryptophan, then you can't make the 5-HTP you need, and you'll fail to produce adequate amounts of serotonin for your brain. To ensure a sufficient supply of 5-HTP, you should eat foods rich in tryptophan (see "Tryptophan," page 100) and possibly take supplements of 5-HTP and/or tryptophan. One strategy would be to begin with a supplement along with an increase in dietary protein, then stop taking the supplement once you reach sufficient levels of serotonin. Often, however, maintenance levels of amino acid supplements are necessary to maintain gains made. If you do not respond well to 5-HTP, tryptophan supplements may be a solution. Every person's needs differ; you (possibly with the help of a health-care practitioner) can find an approach that works best for you.

## How It Works

The antidepressant properties of 5-HTP have been known for decades. In the 1980s, Dr. W. Pöldinger and his colleagues of the Psychiatrische Universitats-klinik in Switzerland found that 5-HTP was as effective as or better than the SSRI fluvoxamine (Luvox) and also caused fewer and less severe side effects. SSRIs and 5-HTP work in different ways, but the end result—at least temporarily—is the same: an increase in the amount of serotonin in the synapse (see figure on page 6). Supplements of 5-HTP are converted into serotonin, thus increasing the brain's supply of the neurotransmitter and allowing more of it to be secreted into the synapse where it has its effect. Once the serotonin is secreted into the synapse and affects the receptors of the adjoining neuron, most of it is taken back up into the original neuron to be used again. The SSRI blocks this reuptake (hence the name *specific serotonin reuptake inhibitor*), which allows the serotonin to remain in the synapse for a longer period of time, thereby having an additional effect on the receptors of the adjoining neuron. Taking an SSRI does not result in the production of more serotonin, which is what the brain may need.

The amino acid 5-HTP is effective in the treatment of symptoms that often accompany depression, including anxiety, aggression, binge eating, chronic headache, insomnia, and sleep difficulties. These qualities proved helpful for Barbara, age thirty-eight, who came to me complaining of depression, fatigue, and an uncontrollable craving for sweets. Although she had an early-morning appointment, she looked tired and pale, and hardly ready for her eight-hour shift at a local bank. The results of her initial neurotransmitter test showed decreased levels of serotonin, norepinephrine, dopamine, epinephrine, and PEA.

The first step was to balance her inhibitory system, which meant we needed to raise Barbara's serotonin level. We increased her 5-HTP dosage to 200 mg twice daily fairly rapidly over a week's time, along with 500 mg vitamin C twice daily—this vitamin is needed to convert 5-HTP to serotonin (see chapter 6). We also made modifications to her diet (see chapter 7), recommended she begin a stress-management practice, and advised her to exercise at least four times a week for thirty to forty-five minutes at a time (see chapter 10).

After three weeks, Barbara reported that she felt somewhat

less depressed. It was then time to balance her excitatory system. To do this, we needed to increase her dopamine levels (dopamine is a precursor to norepinephrine and epinephrine), which we did by starting Barbara on tyrosine (an amino acid precursor of dopamine), 500 mg three times a day, while continuing with the 5-HTP. She steadily improved on this plan, and we retested her neurotransmitter levels after three months. By then, all her levels were within the optimal reference range, and we gradually reduced her amino acid therapy until she was able to come off it completely after a few more months. However, she was cautioned that if her symptoms began to recur, it might mean that her neurotransmitters were again out of balance (possibly as a result of stress); she might need a boost of precursor amino acids.

## Dosage and Side Effects

Supplements of 5-HTP are derived from the seedpods of a West African bean plant called *Griffonia simplicifolia*, and are available as capsules and tablets. Oral doses are well absorbed by the body and easily enter the brain.

The effective dose of 5-HTP can range from 50 to 500 mg daily, but it is recommended that you begin at the lower end of the range and increase gradually until you reach a desired effect. Some people feel positive effects from 5-HTP within a day or two of starting treatment. If you take 5-HTP along with other antidepressant agents, including a prescription drug, you may need only 50 mg or less to get desired results. You should work together with your health-care practitioner to identify the dose that is best for you. Also make sure you get enough complementary nutrients (and especially vitamin $B_6$, magnesium, vitamin C, and vitamin B$_3$, or niacin), either in your diet and/or as supplements, because they are needed for the conversion of 5-HTP to serotonin.

Side effects associated with 5-HTP are typically mild. Temporary gastrointestinal complaints, such as mild bloating or stomachache, may occur because of a possible overproduction of serotonin in the gut. These can be improved or eliminated by starting with a low dose, increasing the dose slowly in small increments, and paying attention to signals given by the body.

## TRYPTOPHAN

Tryptophan is an essential amino acid that has proven to be an effective nutritional treatment for depression. Food sources include poultry (especially turkey), bananas, lentils, peanuts, milk, eggs, and meat, but much of the amino acid in these foods does not reach the brain, so tryptophan or 5-HTP supplements may be necessary.

Up until 1989, tryptophan supplements were used widely around the world, including the United States, and were readily available. That's the year the FDA banned the supplement because a contaminated batch of tryptophan resulted in a number of deaths in the United States (see the discussion on page 95). Even though the tryptophan itself was not the cause of the deaths, the FDA ban continued until recently. As of this writing, tryptophan is available without a prescription in the United States, though it is still not widely available in health food stores.

## How It Works

Tryptophan is an effective natural antidepressant because it is used by the brain to produce serotonin. As you see under the heading "5-HTP" in this chapter, tryptophan is a precursor of 5-HTP, which then goes on to produce serotonin. Individuals who do not respond to 5-HTP or who experience side effects may choose tryptophan as an option.

Along with its role in treating depression, tryptophan also helps induce natural sleep and control alcoholism, as well as reduce sensitivity to pain, anxiety, violent behavior, and obsessive-compulsive behavior. In the mid-1980s, researchers at McGill University found that tryptophan, either alone or along with lithium, was effective in balancing the mood of people with bipolar disorder. In a more recent study (2004), experts documented that a deficiency of tryptophan causes a significant increase in anxiety in people with social anxiety disorder.

## Dosage and Side Effects

The recommended starting dose is 500 mg at bedtime, with increases to 1,000 to 2,000 mg or more as needed. Generally, in terms of supplementation, about 500 mg of tryptophan is equivalent to about 50 mg of 5-HTP.

## GABA (GAMMA AMINOBUTYRIC ACID)

If you're thinking, *Isn't GABA a neurotransmitter?* you're right: GABA is an amino acid that functions as a neurotransmitter in the brain. Thus, unlike the other amino acids discussed in this chapter, GABA acts directly on brain neurons. It is not an essential amino acid; it's made in the body from precursors glutamine and then glutamate. Like serotonin, GABA is an inhibitory neurotransmitter that is helpful during the first phase of targeted amino acid precursor therapy to balance the neurotransmitters. GABA activity may be enhanced by taking supplements such as theanine, glutamic acid, and taurine. Some practitioners, however, including Julia Ross in the book *The Mood Cure*, recommend supplements of GABA itself. I also have found GABA itself to be very helpful in some patients.

I used the GABA-enhancing approach with Walter, a forty-nine-year-old civil engineer who came to me complaining of depression, fatigue, lack of sex drive, and a history of migraines. Neurotransmitter testing indicated a need for GABA as well as 5-HTP, so I prescribed a supplement that contained 5-HTP, theanine, and taurine twice daily, while we also worked on changing his diet (he had never been tested adequately for food allergies, which I suspected were a cause of his migraines) and establishing stress-management and exercise programs. Walter was scheduled to come back to see me three weeks after his initial visit, but he missed it because he had to make an emergency trip to take care of some family business.

When Walter returned six weeks after his initial visit, he reported that he felt much better: His depression had greatly improved, despite having to deal with some anxious moments with his family; his sex drive had returned; and he hadn't had a migraine in two months, while he'd typically had one every four to six weeks. He continued on the previously prescribed supplements, and added precursors for excitatory neurotransmitters. Based on IgG allergy test results, which showed that he had a high level of IgG antibodies to eggs and oranges, I also recommended a trial off eggs and oranges. Walter continues to do well on a maintenance dose of his supplements, a sensible eating plan (see chapter 7), and a daily walking program.

## How It Works

As an inhibitory neurotransmitter, GABA inhibits excessive cell activity and blocks the transmission of signals from one cell to another. This important function helps block anxiety and stress-related impulses in the brain and helps prevent hyperactivity. When there is enough GABA in the brain, activity is more even. Supplementation with GABA-enhancing supplements and/or GABA itself may also enhance sex drive and reduce nighttime urination.

## Dosage and Side Effects

Perhaps one of the best-known advocates of GABA for the treatment of depressive disorders is actress Margot Kidder, who has shared her personal story of recovery from bipolar disorder using natural substances. In an article she wrote for AlternativeMentalHealth.com, she noted that GABA levels are depleted in both the manic and depressed states of bipolar disorder, as is serotonin, another inhibitory neurotransmitter. Ms. Kidder also shared her recipe for success in her fight against bipolar disorder, which includes a daily program of GABA (500 mg), tyrosine, glutamine, taurine, tryptophan, and various nutrients. Other nutrients that help in the production of GABA are inositol, niacinamide, magnesium, vitamin $B_6$, and vitamin C (see chapter 6 for more information about these and other nutrients).

GABA supplements are available as tablets, capsules, and powder. Typical starting doses are 100 to 750 mg two to three times per day. Sublingual tablets that dissolve under the tongue or in the mouth are absorbed into the system more quickly. For some people, dosages in the 500-to-750 mg range cause daytime drowsiness, so lower doses may be more appropriate. Generally, I recommend starting low and increasing slowly for most supplements. If you experience sleepiness or an impaired ability to think or function, the dosage should be reduced or the supplement discontinued. While taking GABA, be aware that any alcohol or other substances that promote relaxation may increase the likelihood of excessive drowsiness.

## GLUTAMINE

Glutamine is a nonessential amino acid that increases the concentration of GABA, the main inhibitory neurotransmitter of the brain and the brain's natural tranquilizer. Significant amounts of glutamine are necessary in the brain to support the complex process of GABA production. If glutamine levels are low, supplementation can not only relieve depression but also alleviate fatigue, speed healing, and reduce cravings for alcohol and other addictive substances such as sugar by a variety of mechanisms. Glutamine is also the precursor of glutamic acid, which neutralizes excess ammonia in the brain, thus improving its molecular environment. In addition, glutamine also may be used as a fuel, like glucose (body sugar), by the brain.

Unlike other cells in the body, brain cells are unable to use fatty acids for fuel and therefore need a constant supply of glucose to function. As you will subsequently see, low-blood-sugar reactions may lead to all kinds of brain reactions, including loss of consciousness. Glutamine is the only other substance besides glucose that may be used as a fuel by the brain.

## How It Works

Glutamine has no trouble passing through the blood–brain barrier. Once in the brain, it is converted (with the help of vitamin $B_6$) to glutamic acid, which in turn may be converted to GABA, thus increasing GABA concentration in the brain. The process is:

### Glutamine → Glutamic acid → GABA

This may prompt you to ask, "Why not take glutamic acid if your GABA levels are low?" Even though glutamic acid is available in supplement form, it does not cross the blood–brain barrier as easily as does glutamine, so the latter is often the supplement of choice to raise GABA levels.

While you might think that amino acid therapy for depression would be most beneficial when it's working in the brain, you would be only partly right. As I mentioned in chapter 2, the health of your gastrointestinal tract is critical for mental as well as physical well-being, and glutamine plays a role here as well. Glutamine helps keep the stomach and intestinal tract healthy by nourishing the cells that line these organs. In addition, glutamine nourishes the immune system. Thus, this amino acid can also help protect the gastrointestinal tract against leaky gut (discussed in chapter 2) and improve immune functioning.

## Dosage and Side Effects

Glutamine is available alone in tablets, capsules, and powders, and as a component in several nutritional formulations. As a therapeutic dose, 500 mg twice daily is often recommended, but much larger doses can be used in selected cases. In rare cases, however, doses of 2,000 mg or greater per day may cause overstimulation and result in restlessness, insomnia, and anxiety.

If you tend to be hypersensitive to monosodium glutamate (MSG) or glutamate (which is composed of two salts of glutamic acid), use of glutamine—which may be converted in the body to glutamic acid or glutamate—can cause headache, chest pain, and other side effects. If you have any of these sensitivities, glutamine should be used with caution.

## PHENYLALANINE

Phenylalanine is an essential amino acid found in many protein foods, including meats, soybeans, poultry, fish, nuts, seeds, dairy products, and the artificial sweetener aspartame (don't consider the latter a source of this amino acid!). However, deficiencies can result from the impact of environmental stressors, poor diet, and other factors, leading to depression, memory difficulties, and decreased sexual energy. Supplementation may reverse these conditions.

Phenylalanine (or tyrosine, an amino acid also discussed in this chapter) is necessary for the production of the excitatory neurotransmitters dopamine and norepinephrine. The sequence goes like this:

**Phenylalanine** → **Tyrosine** → **Dopa** → **Dopamine** → **Norepinephrine**

If your test results show you have a dopamine and/or norepinephrine deficiency, phenylalanine may be helpful.

## How It Works

Phenylalanine occurs in two forms. D-phenylalanine or DPA inhibits the metabolism of endorphins. L-phenylalanine is the form that takes part in the conversion to tyrosine, dopa, dopamine, and norepinephrine described above. A combination of the two forms is available in a supplement known as DL-phenylalanine or DLPA. DLPA is effective in treating depression and in reducing pain through the various possible mechanisms mentioned here. Both D- and L-phenylalanine can be converted in the body to a neurochemical called phenylethylamine, or PEA. It is believed that a deficiency of PEA, which aids in the release of norepinephrine and dopamine, is one cause of depression. In fact, studies show that PEA is low in some people who are depressed. Since PEA is not available as a supplement, phenylalanine supplements—as L-phenylalanine or DLPA—are the next best thing.

## Dosage and Side Effects

Phenylalanine is available in capsules and powders. A typical starting dose is 375 to 500 mg of L-phenylalanine one to three times daily. It works best if taken on an empty stomach about thirty minutes before a meal and along with a B-complex supplement.

If you have high blood pressure or are prone to anxiety or panic attacks, DLPA may aggravate these conditions. Do not take DLPA if you are pregnant or breast-feeding, or if you have malignant melanoma or phenylketonuria. Phenylketonuria is a genetic disease in babies who lack an enzyme for converting phenylalanine to tyrosine. Unless these babies are given a diet free of phenylalanine during the first year or two of life, they will develop severe mental retardation and die. If, however, this special diet is given, new enzymes develop a year or two later and foods containing phenylalanine can be given. Some folks with a milder form of this genetic abnormality have difficulty tolerating phenylalanine. If you seem to have reactions when you take phenylalanine, you may have a mild form of this genetic abnormality and should avoid the substance; use the supplement tyrosine instead.

Side effects from L-phenylalanine include high blood pressure, agitation, insomnia, and anxiety. Those associated with DLPA include heartburn, nausea, and headache. Numbness, tingling, and other signs of nerve damage may occur if you take more than 1,500 mg daily. Use caution if you are taking DLPA along with prescription antidepressants or stimulants, because it may aggravate side effects of the drugs.

Some research shows that DLPA is effective when used along with SAMe or the herbal antidepressant St.-John's-wort. When combined with the latter, levels of both norepinephrine (from the DLPA) and serotonin (from St.-John's-wort) are increased.

## TYROSINE

Most protein foods contain tyrosine, a nonessential amino acid that may also be manufactured in the body from phenylalanine, as shown on page 107. Since tyrosine leads to the production of dopamine and norepinephrine, tyrosine may be helpful when there is a deficiency of one or both of these neurotransmitters. In addition to being a precursor neurotransmitter, tyrosine is also a precursor for thyroid hormones and epinephrine (which is formed from norepinephrine) in the adrenal medulla, the central portion of the adrenal glands. If your depression is associated with an imbalance of these hormones, tyrosine may help you. Tyrosine is also found in soy products, chicken, turkey, fish, peanuts, almonds, avocados, bananas, milk, cheese, lima beans, and sesame seeds.

### Dosage and Side Effects

Tyrosine is available as a powder and in capsules. A typical dose for depression is 500 mg taken two to three times daily, thirty to sixty minutes before meals, but higher doses may be used. Tyrosine is clearly a case of *a little goes a long way*. It's been shown that small doses of the amino acid are more effective in increasing neurotransmitter levels in the brain than are large doses; the latter inhibit the enzyme tyrosine hydroxylase, which converts tyrosine to neurotransmitters.

Vitamin $B_6$, folic acid, and copper should be taken along with tyrosine, because they are necessary for the conversion of tyrosine into the neurotransmitters. Too high a dose of tyrosine can cause irritability and overstimulation.

If you take levodopa while using tyrosine, it may interfere

with the absorption of the amino acid. Do not take tyrosine if you are using a monoamine oxidase inhibitor (MAOI) such as selegiline (Deprenyl, Eldepryl) or isocarboxazid (Marplan); this combination can cause a rise in blood pressure. Consult with your health-care practitioner before taking tyrosine if you have hyperthyroidism or glaucoma or if you are taking methylphenidate (Concerta, Metadate, Ritalin). Generally, you should avoid tyrosine if you have high blood pressure, cancer, or muscular dystrophy, or if you are subject to heart palpitations or migraines.

Recently, some practitioners like myself have begun to use the acetylated form (an acetic acid group is added to tyrosine) of tyrosine called N-acetyltyrosine, because it appears to enter the brain more easily. The dosage needed is generally in the range of 300 mg to 600 mg daily.

## MUCUNA PRURIENS

Another supplement I need to mention here is *Mucuna pruriens*, a climbing woody vine whose seeds are rich in L-dopa, the immediate precursor of dopamine (see the production sequence on page 107). I sometimes use this supplement, along with tyrosine, to increase excitatory amino acids such as dopamine and norepinephrine.

## OTHER AMINO ACIDS

### Cysteine

Cysteine is a sulfur-containing nonessential amino acid that can be made in the body from the essential amino acid methionine. Cysteine plays several roles in relieving depression. One, it aids in detoxification of the body by enhancing the biosynthesis of glutathione, a potent antioxidant that is essential for the liver to perform detoxification. Because cysteine is a chelator (it binds metals to itself so they can be eliminated from the body), it helps protect the body from excess copper and other harmful metals. (See chapter 8.) Two, it is a component of tyrosine hydroxylase, an enzyme that is necessary for the conversion of tyrosine to dopa, dopamine, and norepinephrine. Three, it helps preserve SAMe, which is required for the synthesis of some neurotransmitters.

If you supplement with cysteine, the best form to take is N-acetylcysteine (NAC), which more readily crosses the blood–brain barrier and is more bioavailable. The supplement cysteine is converted in the body to cystine, which is not active.

## Theanine

Theanine is a free-form amino acid that is derived from glutamic acid and is found naturally in green tea and some types of mushrooms. Although its impact on mood has not been studied extensively, the *Physicians' Desk Reference* reports it may have mood-modulating effects. This would appear to be true, because theanine enhances GABA activity as well as regulating the excretion of serotonin, dopamine, epinephrine, and norepinephrine, and can be used to decrease glutamate activity. It helps produce a relaxed state without causing daytime drowsiness.

In one small study of theanine, female volunteers aged eighteen through twenty-two were given either placebo, 50 mg of theanine, or 200 mg of theanine once a week. Anxiety levels were analyzed by measuring their brain waves sixty minutes after each dose. Volunteers who took theanine had significantly greater production of alpha wave activity—an indication of relaxation—than those who took placebo. There was more alpha wave activity, and thus greater relaxation, among volunteers who took the higher dose of theanine.

How does theanine work? Once ingested, it is carried across the blood–brain barrier and into the central nervous system. There it binds to different types of excitatory glutamate receptors on nerve cells. It also stimulates the release of GABA, the main inhibitory neurotransmitter that counterbalances the stimulatory effects of glutamate. Theanine encourages the body to make its own GABA rather than relying on an outside source.

Theanine also triggers the release of dopamine, which contributes to a sense of well-being and pleasure, and norepinephrine. Its effect on serotonin is more uncertain. One study indicated that theanine did not affect serotonin levels, two studies reported that it decreased levels, and a fourth stated that serotonin levels increased in some areas of the brain. However, we use theanine together with 5-HTP frequently with excellent results.

Recommended doses of theanine vary from 100 to 600 mg or more daily, depending on the level of anxiety and difficulty sleeping, because this amino acid has been shown to help induce sleep.

### Histidine

The essential amino acid histidine is sometimes used when histamine is believed to be low in the brain. Histamine is a neurotransmitter that plays a role in helping the release of excitatory neurotransmitters. Its precursor is histidine, which can be given in doses of 500 mg or more before meals.

## SAMe

In 1999, a new treatment for depression hit the market in the United States. S-adenosylmethionine, more commonly known as SAMe, is not an amino acid found in food, but rather an amino acid intermediate formed in the body and found in every cell. It is synthesized as a result of a reaction between the essential amino acid methionine and the major energy compound of the body called ATP, or adenosine triphosphate.

SAMe has been available in Europe since 1975 and underwent decades of extensive study there before it was introduced in the United States as a supplement. Researchers found that SAMe is not only significantly better than placebo in relieving depressive symptoms, but also is comparable to conventional tricyclic antidepressants, and with minimal side effects. In addition, it helps the body eliminate old neurotransmitters, a process that may help new neurotransmitters bind to receptor sites and thus improve their levels in the brain and facilitate cell communication.

SAMe is a methyl donor, which means it donates methyl groups to other substances (see "Methylation" in the introduction to part 2). It also helps regulate different hormones and neurotransmitters, including serotonin, dopamine, and melatonin.

A typical starting dose of SAMe for depression is 400 mg four times per day or 800 mg twice daily (it comes in 200 mg or 400 mg tablets). Once a response occurs, usually within three weeks, the dosage may gradually be reduced to 800 mg or even 400 mg daily based on depressive symptoms. The form that is most bioavailable (easily used by the body) is called butanedisulfonate and comes in enteric-coated tablets. Side effects are infrequent, generally mild, and may include dry mouth, nausea, restlessness, and elation. I recommend taking a B-complex supplement along with SAMe to help prevent a rise in homocysteine levels. (See the discussion of methylation at the beginning of part 2.) If you have bipolar disorder, SAMe should be used only under the strict supervision of a health-care practitioner.

## Taurine

Taurine is a nonessential amino acid that serves several important functions in the body, including acting as a neuromodulator, by helping to prevent overactivity by the excitatory neurotransmitters, which may lead to cell death. In this way, taurine is like the amino acids GABA and glycine, which also help to calm an excited brain. Taurine, as a component of bile, assists in the digestion of fats and fat-soluble vitamins, such as vitamins A, D, and E, and in the optimal use of calcium, magnesium, and sodium. It can be derived from food (good sources are cheese, pork, oatmeal flakes, milk, and fowl), but it is also manufactured in the body from two other amino acids, cysteine and methionine, and aided in the process by vitamin $B_6$.

While a sufficient amount of taurine in the body can help maintain a sense of calm, deficiency can lead to anxiety, hyperactivity, and overall brain dysfunction. Clinical studies conducted by researchers at the Shealy Institute for Comprehensive Health Care in Springfield, Missouri, for example, indicate that at least 78 percent of chronically depressed individuals have a taurine deficiency.

Low levels or a deficiency of taurine can be found in people for many different reasons. Women, for example, may have low levels if they are taking estrogen, because this hormone inhibits the production of taurine in the liver. Individuals who have diabetes have an increased need for taurine. If you use insulin and are considering taking taurine, first talk to your physician, who may decrease your insulin dose while you take this amino acid. Chronic or long-term stress and alcohol use increase your need for taurine as well. Taurine is also closely bound to zinc and manganese; thus, a deficiency in one or both of these elements can interfere with the body's ability to utilize taurine.

I have found that the supplement magnesium taurate is extremely beneficial for patients who have anxiety and palpitations, often providing drastic improvement after just a few doses. The preparation I use has 125 mg magnesium bound to about 440 mg taurine, and I prescribe one to eight capsules daily in divided dosages. Higher doses of magnesium may cause loose stools, necessitating lowering the dose.

One caveat associated with taurine is for those who have gastritis or ulcers. Because this amino acid supplement can promote production of stomach acid, it should be used with caution by individuals with these disorders.

## AMINO ACID THERAPY AND MEDICATION

Unlike some conventional psychiatrists and also some alternative practitioners, I believe that the use of drugs and amino acid therapy need not be mutually exclusive. In fact, for some patients the simultaneous use of these two approaches is an effective strategy. One strong argument for simultaneous use is that the addition of amino acids to a treatment program that includes SSRIs helps to prevent long-term depletion of neurotransmitter levels, because the amino acids build and maintain these levels.

The concurrent use of amino acid therapy and medication follows the same principle as the use of amino acid therapy alone: to bring some balance first to the inhibitory neurotransmitter system, then to the excitatory system, and then to create a balance between the two. Before adding amino acid therapy to your medication regimen, your health-care practitioner may want to determine your biochemical profile and identify which neurotransmitters need to be brought into balance (as discussed in chapter 3), then select the amino acids that will work synergistically to make this happen, along with the medications you are currently taking. Amino acid therapy can be used along with SSRIs (Prozac, Zoloft, Effexor, Lexapro, Paxil), benzodiazepines (Valium, Xanax), tricyclics (desipramine, Aventyl), stimulants (Concerta, Provigil, Ritalin), and anticonvulsants (Neurontin, valproic acid), but not with monoamine oxidase inhibitors (Marplan, Nardil, Parnate), because with this class of drugs, it is much more difficult to control side effects such as high blood pressure. Adding amino acid therapy to a program that includes psychotropic drugs must be done slowly and carefully with the help of a physician familiar with both classes of substances.

One great benefit of amino acid therapy is that it can lead to increased effectiveness of certain medications and hormones. For example, I have had patients come to me who have been on an SSRI such as sertraline (Zoloft) or venlafaxine (Effexor) for more than six months, complaining that the drugs "just don't work." Prolonged use of these antidepressants does indeed lead to depletion of serotonin and norepinephrine stores in the brain (see chapter 12). However, the addition of appropriate amino acid therapy not only increases the effectiveness of the drugs but can also result in some patients weaning themselves off the drugs completely, a goal I always strive for in my practice. Amino acid therapy also increases the body's sensitivity to hormone replacement therapy and results in a decreased need for the hormones.

Because amino acid therapy typically enhances an individual's sensitivity to certain medications by improving the signaling system in the body, some people experience "overdosing side effects." These symptoms can be eliminated quickly by reducing the medication dosage, which should be done under your physician's care.

## THE BOTTOM LINE

Amino acid therapy is a critical component of an effective treatment plan for depression. By providing the body with the precursors it needs to produce neurotransmitters associated with depressed mood, you correct the imbalance underlying depression rather than just its symptoms. You also have the added benefit of avoiding or greatly reducing your exposure to side effects associated with the use of antidepressants.

## Chapter 5

# Make the Most of Essential Fatty Acids and Other Fats

One of the most common nutritional imbalances present in the American diet is of the essential fatty acids: the omega-3s and omega-6s. These vital nutrients are found in high concentrations in the brain, where they play major roles in regulating mood and maintaining proper nerve function. When essential fatty acid stores are out of balance—a situation that is true of most Americans—the brain is unable to properly process neurotransmitters, which has a negative effect on mood.

The impact of essential fatty acids on mood and mood-related symptoms is so significant that it warrants its own chapter. In my experience, fatty acid supplementation has been helpful in most depressed patients. You'll learn all about these special nutrients in this chapter and how to add them to your diet.

Enthusiasm about monitoring essential fatty acids should not overshadow the importance of regulating other fats; they, too, have an impact on mood. Thus we also take a brief look at the role of saturated and unsaturated fats in depression and mood.

So now it's time to pull out the Symptom Profile from chapter 3 that lists the characteristics of fat and fatty acid imbalance and see how you fared. If you are like most Americans, you are drawing some parallels. Read on!

## THE FAT STORY

Americans have a love–hate relationship with fat: Consumers fill their shopping carts with foods that are touted as low-fat, no-fat, or fat-free, yet approximately 65 percent of adults in the United States are overweight. Consumers are often the target of conflicting reports about the virtues of fat consumption, on the one hand, and its detrimental effects on the other. The truth is, some fats are essential to optimal health, while a few others are harmful. If you learn the differences between them and how to include the beneficial ones while reducing your consumption of the rest, you'll enjoy not only better physical health but enhanced mental and emotional health as well.

### Types of Fat

Fats, also known as lipids, are mainly present in food as triglycerides, substances that are made by the body from the fat and carbohydrates you eat. Triglycerides are composed of a three-carbon molecule called glycerol attached to three fatty acids. Fatty acids consist of a chain of carbon atoms attached to one another by single or double bonds. Except for the two end carbons, each carbon is attached to one or two hydrogen atoms. At one end of the fatty acid is an acid group attached to two atoms of oxygen. At the other end, the last carbon (or omega carbon) is attached to three hydrogen atoms (so it is a methyl group).

A saturated fatty acid is called *saturated* because no more hydrogen atoms can be added to it; with an *unsaturated* fatty acid, more hydrogen atoms can be added. *Monounsaturated* fatty acids and *polyunsaturated* fatty acids are types of unsaturated fatty acids, while *omega-3* and *omega-6* fatty acids are a subgroup of polyunsaturated fatty acids known as essential fatty acids. Finally, the other class of fatty acids we will concern ourselves with is *trans-fatty acids*, which are man-made and interfere with the normal functioning of fatty acids. All of this terminology will be helpful as we discuss fats and fatty acids.

The fatty acids can be any combination of saturated (including animal fat, butter, lard), monounsaturated (found most commonly in olive oil), polyunsaturated (flaxseed oil, soybean oil, fish oils), or trans-fatty acids (polyunsaturated fatty acids that have undergone hydrogenation; see page 133). If the fat is hard, then most of the fatty acids on the triglyceride are saturated and/or contain trans-fatty acids. If the fat is liquid or soft, then most of the fatty acids are polyunsaturated. If you look at the ingredient label on many food items, you will see a figure for total fat and a breakdown of the different fatty acids— saturated, monounsaturated, polyunsaturated, and/or trans-fatty acids. As of January 1, 2006, food manufacturers were required to provide trans-fat information on food labels.

## Benefits of Dietary Fat

Although the word *fat* may conjure up many negative thoughts and images for some people, fat serves several critical functions in human health. One, at 9 calories per gram, it is a very concentrated source of energy. Two, fat is a basic component in all cell membranes and critical for cell function. This is especially important in the brain, which is more than 60 percent fat. That's because the brain cells are covered by a fat-rich myelin sheath.

Three, specific types of polyunsaturated fats known as essential fatty acids, which I discuss in detail below, are necessary for the production of prostaglandins, short-acting hormone-like substances that are important in the regulation of, among other things, nerve transmission (fats play a critical role as messengers), inflammation, pain, water retention, allergic reactions, and hormone synthesis. In contrast to endocrine hormones such as thyroid, adrenal, or sex hormones—which exist for long periods of time, travel in the bloodstream, and act on distant organs—prostaglandins do not enter the bloodstream; they act locally on cells where they are formed and are metabolized in seconds or less.

## ESSENTIAL FATTY ACIDS

I begin with the fats that have the most impact on mood, the essential fatty acids, specifically omega-3 and omega-6. These fats belong to a group of fatty acids called polyunsaturated fatty acids, or PUFAs. They are "essential" because they are necessary for health but cannot be manufactured by the body. Therefore, your food and supplement choices are critical because they can help you achieve and maintain an optimal balance of omega-3 and omega-6, which together play a crucial role in balanced mood, hormone synthesis, brain function and development, nerve transmission, and energy production.

Both omega-3 and omega-6 fatty acids come in several forms. We'll look at each of these fatty acids separately to see how they operate in the body and what role they play in determining mood. Then I'll talk about why it's critical for mental health to maintain a balance between these two categories of fatty acids.

## Omega-6 Fatty Acids

The omega-6 fatty acids are sometimes billed as "bad guys," but that is not the case when they are consumed in reasonable amounts in balance with omega-3 fatty acids. To help you understand what happens when you consume omega-6 fatty acids, refer to the figure below, which I explain here.

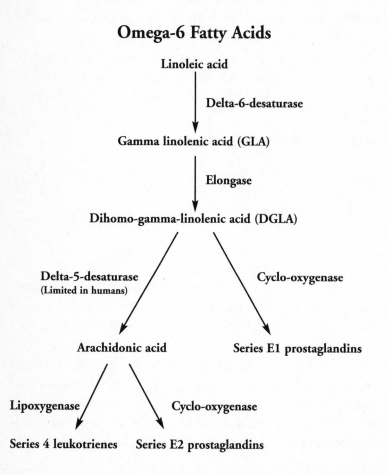

### Omega-6 Fatty Acids

Linoleic acid

Delta-6-desaturase

Gamma linolenic acid (GLA)

Elongase

Dihomo-gamma-linolenic acid (DGLA)

Delta-5-desaturase
(Limited in humans)

Cyclo-oxygenase

Arachidonic acid

Series E1 prostaglandins

Lipoxygenase

Cyclo-oxygenase

Series 4 leukotrienes

Series E2 prostaglandins

Much of the omega-6 fatty acids consumed by Americans are in the form of linoleic acid, which is found in most vegetable oils, such as corn, safflower, soybean, and sunflower, as well as margarines and in many processed foods. An enzyme called delta-6-desaturase converts the linoleic acid into gamma linolenic acid (GLA), which in turn metabolizes into dihomo-gamma-linolenic acid (DGLA). Action by an enzyme called cyclo-oxygenase turns some DGLA into series E1 prostaglandins, substances that help decrease inflammation, reduce pain, and provide cardiovascular benefits by relaxing blood vessels and lowering blood pressure. When another enzyme called delta-5-desaturase acts on DGLA, the result is arachidonic acid, which is abundant in the brain and essential to its function. This acid also reacts with cyclo-oxygenase and converts to the series E2 prostaglandins, which, in excess, promote depression, cause inflammation, and make platelets stick together excessively.

As the figure shows, arachidonic acid converts to series E2 prostaglandins. While there are several conversions necessary to transform linoleic acid into arachidonic acid (and these reactions take place only to a limited extent in humans) and then to series E2 prostaglandins, those steps are bypassed if you consume foods rich in arachidonic acid, which include egg yolks, most meats, and other animal-based foods. Thus, when you consider that the standard American diet consists mainly of animal-based foods and foods that contain or are prepared with vegetable oils, it is clear why omega-6 consumption tends to be greater than that of omega-3 fatty acids, which are found primarily in fish and in a few other foods (see "Omega-3 Fatty Acids," below).

You can also get GLA directly by consuming special plant oils—borage, black currant seed, and evening primrose oils. These are usually taken in a supplement form to help fight inflammation. Fortunately, much of the GLA taken as a supplement can be converted into DGLA, which is then transformed into series E1 prostaglandins in the presence of vitamins $B_3$, $B_6$, and C, and the minerals magnesium and zinc.

## Omega-3 Fatty Acids

The modern Western diet is generally depleted of omega-3 fatty acids. This is a critical issue, as omega-3s are highly concentrated in the brain and play a critical role in mood, behavior, and cognitive function. In fact, about 25 percent of the dry weight of the brain is composed of omega-3s. These fatty acids are key components of nerve cell membranes and help nerve cells communicate with each other. If you are deficient in these essential elements, your brain cells malfunction and you are much more likely to become depressed. Conversely, numerous studies have shown that when omega-3 supplements are taken, people who are depressed improve significantly. Various studies also show that fish consumption is associated with lower incidence of depression.

Researchers have found that serotonin and dopamine levels and activity are altered in animals with omega-3 deficiency, and that these findings are very similar to those seen in autopsy studies of human depression. Other results of an omega-3 deficiency are a decrease in blood flow to the brain and a 35 percent reduction in a brain chemical called phosphatidyl serine, which has some antidepressant activity.

Omega-3 fatty acids also appear to have a grip on your heart. In a letter published in the *Archives of General Psychiatry*, several prominent physicians, including Andrew Stoll, MD, an expert on essential fatty acids and author of *The Omega-3 Connection*, suggest that a low level of omega-3 fatty acids is the "missing link" that may explain why individuals with major depression are at a higher risk for developing and dying from heart disease than those who have normal levels of this nutrient.

A deficiency of omega-3 fatty acids also may be instrumental in postpartum depression in women: Omega-3 preferentially goes to the fetus over the mother, because it is so essential for proper brain development. With each pregnancy, delivery, and breast-feeding, a mother's level of docosahexaenoic acid (DHA), an omega-3 fatty acid, becomes lower and lower, which can result in postpartum depression. Other nutrients such as iodine may also play a role in postpartum depression for similar reasons: Iodine preferentially goes to the fetus, making a borderline-insufficient mother very deficient (see chapters 6 and 9).

What all of this means to you is that you cannot afford to ignore omega-3 fatty acids if you are serious about combating depression. That being said, let's examine the relationships among the three types of omega-3 fatty acids more closely.

## Alpha Linolenic Acid

Alpha linolenic acid, or ALA, is the main plant-based omega-3 fatty acid and the one from which two other omega-3 fatty acids—eicosapentaenoic acid (EPA) and DHA—are derived. All three omega-3 fatty acids are important for optimal health, but they are not all equally readily available from the foods you eat.

For example, when you consume foods that contain ALA, your body converts some of it into EPA and DHA. This conversion isn't very efficient, however. Some research suggests that in healthy people, only 5 to 10 percent of ALA is converted to EPA, while only 2 to 5 percent is transformed into DHA. More recent studies indicate these numbers are closer to 21 percent and 9 percent, respectively.

In either case, the conversion rates are less than ideal. Thus, to help ensure that you get an adequate supply of EPA and DHA, the best sources are foods that already contain these essential fatty acids (see page 127), which enable your body to bypass ALA conversion. If those EPA and DHA sources are not to your liking, you should consume sources of ALA that are highest in ALA. By far the highest concentration is in flaxseed oil (50 percent). Walnut oil has about 13 percent, and soybean oil about 5 percent. For most of my patients, I recommend freshly ground or vacuum-packed organic flaxseed and/or organic flaxseed oil at daily dosages of 1 to 2 tablespoons of either or both (1 tablespoon of flaxseed oil would be equivalent to about 8 to 10 capsules of flaxseed oil, 1,000 mg each).

Once EPA and DHA have been converted from ALA, they are metabolized into series E3 prostaglandins. These hormone-like substances help control the levels of the damaging series E2 prostaglandins that are the result of the conversion of omega-6 fatty acids to arachidonic acid. The E3 series also help reduce inflammation and pain associated with inflammatory conditions such as rheumatoid arthritis, Raynaud's phenomenon, and lupus.

## Eicosapentaenoic Acid and Docosahexaenoic Acid

EPA and DHA are released in the body as the result of the breakdown of ALA. They can also be obtained directly from certain foods, namely fatty fish such as tuna, salmon, herring, sardines, and rainbow trout, among others. Although both of these omega-3 fatty acids are essential for optimal health, EPA is the more prominent of the two for most psychiatric conditions and has been studied more than DHA.

For example, a recent study conducted in England showed that depressed individuals who had not responded to traditional prescription drugs such as SSRIs and tricyclic antidepressants improved significantly when given 1 g per day of EPA for twelve weeks. Another study showed that EPA improved symptoms in people with depressive disorder who were taking lithium. In this study, it was unclear whether EPA augmented the effect of lithium or had antidepressant effects on its own.

In studies of DHA, it's been shown that low levels of the fatty acid in mother's milk and low seafood consumption are associated with higher rates of postpartum depression. Low levels of DHA have also been associated with major depression in people who have acute coronary syndrome.

## How Much Omega-3 Do You Need?

The jury is still out on the ideal amount of omega-3 people should include in their diet and/or supplement program. I find that, like other components of my approach to treatment of depression, the amount a person needs is highly individual, and so it may take several tries at different doses until the best one is found.

- Generally, I prescribe from 1 to 6 g of fish oil, taken in divided doses, depending on the individual's needs, using supplements free of mercury.
- According to the American Heart Association (AHA), some studies indicate that daily intake of 0.5 to 1.8 g of EPA plus DHA, either from fatty fish or supplements, significantly reduces the risk of death from heart disease.
- The AHA also suggests that total daily intake of ALA could be 1.5 to 3 g and recommends that people without coronary heart disease should eat at least two servings of fish (preferably fatty fish) per week, while those with coronary heart disease should get 1 g of EPA/DHA per day from fish and/or supplements. However, I am concerned about the mercury intake when a person eats fish twice a week, unless the fish are chosen carefully and the person's mercury level is monitored.
- See "The Scoop on Fish Oil Supplements" on page 131 for hints on getting the omega-3s you need.

## The Omega-6/Omega-3 Imbalance

Do headache, fatigue, itchy skin, constipation, poor appetite, slowed metabolism, or brittle nails accompany your depression? You, like millions of other Americans, could be living with an imbalance in essential fatty acids. Historically, humans consumed a diet that was believed to be about equal in omega-3 and omega-6 content. Over the millennia, and especially over the past seventy to eighty years, our consumption of omega-3s has declined dramatically. This is particularly true in the United States, where in recent decades omega-3 intake has fallen by about 80 percent, according to Dr. Donald Rudin, an expert in essential fatty acids. The reasons behind this decline include the following. See how many are a part of your lifestyle:

- A decline in the consumption of foods that are a good source of omega-3 fatty acids, such as fish, whole grains, and flaxseed.
- An increase in consumption of foods that contain trans-fatty acids (which interfere with the functioning of omega-3 fatty acids), such as margarines, snack foods like potato chips and corn chips, frozen dinners, cookies and crackers, and fast food.
- An increase in consumption of sugary foods. Sugar interferes with fatty acid metabolism.
- Refining of grains and an increase in the consumption of processed-grain foods, which are stripped of their omega-3 fatty acids.
- An increase in the prevalence of nutritional deficiencies. Some nutrients, such as vitamin $B_6$, are necessary for fatty acid metabolism.

- An increase in the use of pharmaceutical drugs, many of which deplete the body of nutrients and fatty acids.
- Digestive problems.
- Infant formulas, which have previously had insufficient fatty acids, though some essential fatty acids have recently been added to US formulas.

In addition, you can throw in the facts that the body's ability to use essential fatty acids declines with age, and that stress has a negative impact on the conversion of essential fatty acids to prostaglandins.

Along with a decline in the consumption of omega-3 fatty acids, the intake of omega-6 fatty acids (often in a harmful form, such as margarine containing trans-fatty acids) has increased, with the result being an unhealthy ratio of omega-6 to omega-3 fatty acids in the diet. According to an international panel of experts on essential fatty acids, the optimal ratio of omega-6 to omega-3 is about 1:1; Dr. Stoll and also Dr. Yehuda from Israel (who has researched these ratios) prefer 4:1, yet the typical American diet is closer to 25:1 or 30:1. In these studies, moreover, many of the fatty acids that are counted as omega-6 are actually trans-fatty acids, which do not function as omega-6 or omega-3. Thus, many Americans, especially those who eat a lot of fast food and highly processed food, have excessive amounts of trans-fatty acids and may actually be deficient in both omega-6 and omega-3 fatty acids.

Studies show that a deficiency of omega-3 fatty acids and an imbalance of omega-6 to omega-3 fatty acids increase the risk for depression. It's been shown, in fact, that among people hospitalized for depression, levels of omega-3 fatty acids were low and the ratio of omega-6 to omega-3 was out of balance (they had significantly higher omega-6 levels). In addition, most omega-6 fatty acids promote inflammation, while the omega-3s help reduce inflammation. Thus, a diet high in omega-6s can contribute to the development of conditions such as arthritis, heart disease, stroke, and chronic pain, while a healthy ratio maintains and even improves health.

## The Scoop on Fish Oil Supplements

If you choose to take fish oil supplements as your source of omega-3s, you should follow some guidelines. If you bruise easily, have a bleeding disorder, or are taking anticoagulant or antiplatelet drugs, don't add omega-3 fatty acids unless you're under medical supervision; high amounts of omega-3 fatty acids may increase the risk of bleeding in such cases. It's also believed that people who have diabetes or schizophrenia may be unable to convert ALA to EPA and DHA, so fish oil supplements may be especially important if you have either of these conditions.

---

### What to Look for When Shopping for Fish Oil Supplements

- An omega-3 fatty acid concentration of *at least* 30 percent—preferably higher. The higher the concentration, the fewer capsules you will need to take per day.
- An EPA-to-DHA ratio that favors EPA. Research indicates that EPA is the more active of the two omega-3s when it comes to mood. Most fish oil pills contain an EPA-to-DHA ratio of about 3:2; that is, for example,

360 mg EPA and 240 mg DHA, or 18 percent EPA and 12 percent DHA. However, there are fish oil capsule ratios of EPA to DHA of 4:1 or higher. These may be more effective for mood disorders, according to Dr. Stoll and others.

- Cod liver oil capsules contain both vitamin A and vitamin D, both of which can be quite beneficial. In high doses, however, they are potentially toxic; A and D levels need to be monitored.
- Buy fish oil only from manufacturers who certify that their supplements are free of mercury and other toxins.

Some people experience nausea, excessive belching, fishy odor of the breath, and flatulence when taking fish oil pills, all of which reduce the supplement's appeal. However, highly purified, molecularly distilled fish oil liquid or capsules are less likely to cause these problems. Also, the use of time-released preparations often reduces unpleasant reactions.

## SATURATED FATS

Saturated fats are solid at room temperature and are present in animal sources such as meat, eggs, and dairy foods. Some clinicians regard them as "bad" fats because of reports that they can raise your serum levels of bad cholesterol (LDL, or low-density lipoprotein) and promote the formation of blood clots. They also, however, offer many benefits. For example, saturated fats help raise levels of the "good" cholesterol, high-density lipoprotein (HDL) cholesterol, and are necessary for proper modeling of calcium in the bones. They help conserve omega-3 fatty acids, which are in short supply in most Americans, and some of them support the immune system by fighting bacteria, viruses, and other disease-causing organisms. One type of saturated fat, stearic acid, is the preferred fuel for the heart.

Saturated fats are not essential and, although beneficial, should not be used to the exclusion of essential polyunsaturated fats. Aim for a healthy balance of saturated and unsaturated fats. Sources of saturated fatty acids should be clean, meaning free of hormones, pesticides, antibiotics, and other additives.

## TRANS-FATTY ACIDS

Trans-fatty acids are the synthetic by-product of a chemical process called *hydrogenation*, in which great pressure and heat are used to force hydrogen atoms into the molecules of polyunsaturated fats. This process transforms a liquid vegetable oil into a semisolid state to form shortening and/or margarine. Foods that contain margarine or shortening, such as many baked goods, processed foods, and fast foods, also contain trans-fatty acids.

Trans-fatty acids are damaging to the body. For example, they raise the blood level of LDL (low-density lipoprotein) cholesterol and triglycerides and lower the level of HDL cholesterol. These artificially created fats also block the production and metabolism of DHA, impair the body's ability to transform linoleic acid into GLA, disrupt cell processes, deplete the body of nutrients, and are believed to hinder the production of prostaglandins, all actions that can have a negative effect on mood. Clearly, trans-fats are substances you want to eliminate from your diet as much as possible. In chapter 7, I talk about how to pursue a healthful diet that reduces your intake of these fats and maximizes your consumption of the brain-healthy fats—essential fatty acids.

## THE BOTTOM LINE

Good fats versus bad fats—the discussion seems to never end. When it comes to beating depression and its related symptoms, include essential omega-6 and omega-3 fatty acids in a ratio of approximately 4:1, and include some saturated fatty acids as well. As much as possible, eliminate all hydrogenated fats that contain trans-fatty acids. This is the recipe for balanced mood—and overall health as well.

## Chapter 6

———— ❧ ————

# Lift Your Spirits with Nutrients and Herbs

At this very moment, fifteen trillion nerve cells in your brain are hungry for specific nutrients that they need to function. Deprive your brain of these nutrients—even one—and the result can be devastating. Nutrients are necessary for neuro-transmitter production, hormone secretion, nerve transmission, and cell metabolism. When nutritional imbalances occur, as often happens in today's calorie-rich, nutrient-poor diets, each of these areas can suffer, and the result can be depression, confusion, fatigue, insomnia, loss of sex drive, anxiety, and other symptoms that often accompany mood disorders. When you correct nutrient deficiencies, however, symptoms can be alleviated and mind–body harmony can be restored. In the pages that follow, I explain how you can do just that.

We know, for example, that vitamin $B_6$ is important in the conversion of tryptophan and 5-hydroxytryptophan (5-HTP) to serotonin. Thus, a $B_6$ deficiency could explain why 5-HTP supplements fail to raise serotonin levels in some people, even if they have been taking tryptophan or 5-HTP. This is just one example of why it is important to examine your dietary habits when treating depression, because even one deficiency may be the reason why a particular treatment strategy isn't effective.

In this chapter, we will take a closer look at not only the nutrients but also the herbs that can play a crucial role in relieving depression and improving overall mood. Although I firmly believe that people should get the majority of their nutrients from eating healthful, whole foods, I also know that most individuals need at least a few supplements to achieve optimal nutrition as well as balance in other areas, such as neurotransmitters and hormones. I believe you'll find, as my patients do, that adding certain nutrients and herbs to your lifestyle will not only enhance your mood but pay benefits in physical health as well.

## VITAMINS AND MINERALS AND HOW THEY WORK

I have discussed many biochemical reactions and indicated that vitamins and minerals are important in them, but haven't really explained what they are or how they work in the body. Vitamins are generally small molecules (compared, for example, with large protein molecules) that are necessary for life and health, but cannot be made by the body (with a few exceptions, as discussed in this book). They must be ingested orally from food or nutritional supplements, or injected into the body. All vitamins are *organic* molecules, which means that they all contain carbon atoms. In addition to vitamins, we all need to take in essential minerals via food, nutritional supplements, or injection. Minerals are *inorganic* elements (they do not contain carbon atoms, although they may bind to organic molecules), such as calcium, magnesium, iron, zinc, and chromium.

In the body, vitamins and minerals assist enzymes, specific protein molecules that speed up or catalyze chemical reactions, allowing them to occur quickly. Generally, one specific enzyme catalyzes a specific biochemical reaction in the body. To function, each enzyme requires smaller molecules—namely, a specific vitamin and mineral. This combination of vitamin and mineral is called a *coenzyme* or *cofactor* for that particular enzymatic reaction.

Vitamins and minerals are needed by the body in relatively small amounts (micrograms or milligrams), compared with grams needed for the macronutrients, protein, fats, and carbohydrates. However, if an enzyme is deficient, either because of a genetic abnormality or for another reason, or if an enzyme is damaged (possibly as a result of an environmental toxin, such as mercury), supplying relatively large amounts of the vitamin and/or mineral can help the enzyme to do its job much better. When a person needs a large amount of a specific vitamin, it's known as *vitamin dependency.* Throughout this and other chapters, I frequently recommend doses of vitamins considered by conventional medicine to be excessive. Often, this is because my experience tells me that certain patients have become dependent on specific supplements for optimal functioning. One good example is that women with depression and other symptoms associated with the premenstrual syndrome (PMS) often respond beautifully to relatively high doses of vitamin $B_6$ (100 mg three times daily), along with magnesium (100 mg three times daily) and zinc (25 mg once or twice daily). We will encounter other examples in this book.

Another important issue to understand is the difference

between the recommended daily allowance (RDA) and the optimal dosage of supplements. The RDA for various nutrients reflects the amount of the substance needed to prevent a deficiency disease or condition (such as scurvy in the case of vitamin C, or an enlarged thyroid gland or goiter in the case of iodine) in healthy individuals and is not necessarily the optimal dosage for any specific person. It does not allow for the presence of disease or illness, the level of stress, biochemical individuality, diet, the use of medications, or other factors that can impact a person's need for certain nutrients. The optimal dosage for an individual is often many times the RDA. For your convenience, at the end of this chapter, I present a list of approximate dosage ranges of nutrients for optimal functioning for many folks to prevent and/or treat depression.

## THE B VITAMINS

Although many vitamins and nutrients can influence the mind and mood, various B vitamins are especially critical when it comes to maintaining optimal nerve cell metabolism and function, and thus can have a dramatic effect. Like members of a family, they depend on each other to accomplish their tasks. Indeed, the special synergistic relationship among the B vitamins is demonstrated in the fact that they are available as a B-complex supplement that supplies a balance of the main B vitamins.

How important is this balance? For a twenty-nine-year-old professional musician named Colleen, it proved critical. When she came to see me, she had many of the classic symptoms of depression: low sex drive, insomnia, withdrawal, and irritability. She and her husband, Joshua, had been married for less than a year, and she was taking birth control pills as they did not want to start a family for several years. Because she and Joshua wanted to buy a house before having children, they were both working long hours to save for a down payment, and Colleen had taken a part-time job as a receptionist in addition to playing the piano at various venues around the city. As a result, she was rushing from one job to another, often not finding time to eat or just stopping for what she admitted was "really bad fast food."

Test results revealed that Colleen had low levels of several vitamins and minerals, but most notably $B_6$, $B_{12}$, and folic acid. Deficiencies of these B vitamins are not unusual among women who take birth control pills and/or people who rely heavily on a fast-food diet. I immediately placed Colleen on a high-potency B-complex supplement and we discussed changes to her diet, but she did not want to stop taking birth control. With the addition of the B-complex supplement, modifications to her diet, and participation in stress-management exercises (she started yoga classes), Colleen's depression and its accompanying symptoms improved dramatically within a few weeks. After two months, she said she felt nearly "normal" again.

Not every case is as easy to address as Colleen's, but it does illustrate how a deficiency of just a few B vitamins can significantly impact mood. Even so, Colleen took a B-complex supplement rather than individual supplements of the three B vitamins in which she was deficient, because the goal was not only to eliminate deficiencies but also to achieve a balance. An excess of one B vitamin can lead to a deficiency of another.

We will now take a look at the B vitamins and the interrelationships they have, especially as related to depression and mood disorders.

### Vitamin B₁ (Thiamine)

The brain needs thiamine to metabolize carbohydrates for energy. Low levels of this vitamin can result in fatigue, irritability, memory lapses, insomnia, stomach upset, and loss of appetite. Severe vitamin $B_1$ deficiency, or beriberi, is characterized by loss of appetite with subsequent weight loss, enlargement of the heart, and neuromuscular symptoms such as paresthesia (spontaneous sensations like burning or itching), muscle weakness, general weakness, and foot and wrist droop. Individuals who are most at risk for a serious deficiency include chronic alcoholics, pregnant or nursing women, people who have a chronic illness such as a malabsorption syndrome or liver disease, people who eat mostly fast food and/or junk food, individuals involved with long-term use of loop diuretics, drug addicts, and the elderly.

In one study, vitamin $B_1$ levels were tested in children and adolescents who had severe behavioral disturbances, depression, and anxiety. The vast majority of these children, who ate mainly junk foods, had a vitamin $B_1$ deficiency. They were treated with large doses (several hundred milligrams daily) of vitamin $B_1$ and a reduction in their intake of refined carbohydrates. Within a few months, most of the children improved.

For adults, I usually recommend 10 to 50 mg daily of vitamin $B_1$, although the RDA is much less. I also encourage my patients to eat foods rich in thiamine, such as vegetables, whole grains, nuts, seeds, and legumes.

## Vitamin B$_2$ (Riboflavin)

Riboflavin is necessary for metabolism of essential fatty acids and for enhancing energy production in brain cells. A deficiency is associated with symptoms of depression, especially among women who take oral contraceptives and those who are in their second trimester of pregnancy. I often recommend 10 to 50 mg of riboflavin daily along with foods rich in this vitamin, including whole grains, beans, green leafy vegetables, yogurt, soybeans, and fish.

Many people with depression require vitamin B$_6$. If we give relatively high doses of B$_6$ without vitamin B$_2$, a relative deficiency of vitamin B$_2$ may occur. A symptom associated with B$_2$ deficiency is cheilosis, an inflammation at the corners of the mouth.

## Vitamin B$_3$ (Niacin)

Niacin helps maintain blood glucose levels and energy production. It is also a close relative and component of NADH, another nutrient important in mood (see "NADH," page 142). In contrast with most vitamins, the body can make niacin from tryptophan. If sufficient niacin is present in the diet or as a supplement, more tryptophan may be used to make serotonin, rather than being diverted into making niacin. Low levels of niacin can cause depression, along with agitation, anxiety, and mental fogginess, while chronic deficiency can lead to psychosis and dementia. Severe niacin deficiency causes the disease known as pellagra, characterized by dermatitis, diarrhea, and dementia (the three Ds).

Individuals most at risk of a niacin deficiency are alcoholics, drug addicts, the elderly, and people who have liver disease, diabetes, pancreas disease, stomach ulcer, or an overactive thyroid, or who are under prolonged stress. The recommended therapeutic daily dose of niacin for adults is 25 to 50 mg. However, for some patients with extreme symptoms, as might occur in schizophrenia, much larger doses may be recommended. Food sources include brown rice, whole grains, barley, seeds, peanuts, and almonds.

## NADH

Nicotinamide adenine dinucleotide with hydrogen, or NADH, is a close relative of niacin that exists in all living cells and is especially concentrated in the brain and central nervous system. It has mood-elevating properties, because it stimulates the production of several neurotransmitters, including L-dopa, dopamine, and norepinephrine.

Jorg G. D. Birkmayer, MD, PhD, an authority on NADH, discovered the ability of NADH to reduce symptoms of depression while he was conducting research on people with Parkinson's disease. In his study of more than two hundred depressed patients whom he treated with NADH, 93 percent benefited from the treatment.

Supplementation with NADH may be especially helpful if your depression is related to low dopamine levels or activity, or to a condition that causes Parkinsonian neurological symptoms. The recommended daily dose for adults is 5 to 10 mg. NADH is safe and nontoxic, though in rare cases, high doses may cause anxiety, insomnia, and jitteriness.

## Vitamin B₅ (Pantothenic Acid)

Vitamin $B_5$ plays a role in carbohydrate metabolism, the production of adrenal hormones, and essential fatty acid activity. Individuals who have depression that is related to an imbalance in blood sugar can benefit from taking vitamin $B_5$. Although I consider the optimal daily dose for adults to be about 25 to 50 mg, people who are depressed often benefit most from 100 to 250 mg per day and report improved mood, increased energy, and being more alert. Sometimes even larger doses (1,000 mg to 3,000 mg daily in divided doses) are beneficial in patients with low adrenal function; however, dosages greater than 250 mg may cause insomnia in some patients. You can get your pantothenic acid in avocados, eggs, brown rice, lentils, bananas, soybeans, and mushrooms.

## Vitamin B₆ (Pyridoxine)

Along with folic acid and vitamin $B_{12}$, vitamin $B_6$ is intimately associated with mood. Levels of vitamin $B_6$ are typically low in people who are depressed, especially women who take any form of estrogen. A vitamin $B_6$ deficiency can also be due to inadequate dietary intake, high intake of protein, diseases that cause malabsorption, excessive alcohol use, or an unusually fast metabolism.

Vitamin $B_6$ is necessary for healthy blood, skin, and several critical brain functions. Specifically, it slows the destruction of tryptophan, which in turn enhances serotonin functioning and helps convert tryptophan to serotonin. It also is involved in the production of cysteine and glutathione from homocysteine, plays a role in converting tyrosine to norepinephrine, and works with folic acid to help prevent depletion of SAMe, a substance required for the conversion of norepinephrine to epinephrine.

Depressed patients who are deficient in vitamin $B_6$ typically respond dramatically to supplementation. While a recommended maintenance level for adults is 25 to 50 mg daily, therapeutic doses generally start at 50 mg twice a day for several weeks, followed by 50 mg once daily. Sometimes much larger doses are recommended. The active form of vitamin $B_6$ is pyridoxal-5-phosphate (P5P), which is available as a supplement. It is ten times more potent; thus 10 mg of P5P is equivalent to about 100 mg of pyridoxine.

If you take $B_6$ as a supplement, you should also take magnesium, because they often work together, and use of high doses of $B_6$ without magnesium may result in irritability and anxiety. High doses of $B_6$ (more than 500 mg daily) over long periods of time may result in symptoms of nerve dysfunction, but this is reversible when the $B_6$ is stopped.

Good food sources of pyridoxine include meats, fish (especially salmon and herring), brown rice, cauliflower, spinach, walnuts, eggs, bananas, onions, broccoli, squash, kale, peas, and brussels sprouts.

### Vitamin $B_{12}$ (Cobalamin)

A minute amount of vitamin $B_{12}$ goes a long way, so don't let its low RDA—4 to 6 mcg for adults—fool you. As with folic acid, a $B_{12}$ deficiency alone can cause depression, especially among the elderly. In fact, about 20 percent of older adults do not adequately absorb $B_{12}$ from their intestines, so that they are at risk for a $B_{12}$ deficiency even if they eat foods that contain this vitamin. Yet many physicians don't address this very real, and fortunately easily remedied, cause of depression among older adults.

Sixty-nine-year-old Arlene knows what it's like to have her depression be ignored by her doctor. A retired teacher and a widow, she lived alone in an apartment in a retirement community, where she had many friends and access to a variety of activities. Yet Arlene was depressed, finding it increasingly difficult to leave her apartment. She was also experiencing some confusion, memory loss, and fatigue, and her daughter, Ellie, feared her mother was developing Alzheimer's disease. Yet these are also symptoms of a vitamin $B_{12}$ deficiency, which we discovered when Ellie brought her mother to our facility.

I wasn't the first doctor Arlene had visited. She had expressed her concerns to her primary physician, who dismissed her complaints and told her to "socialize more." After talking with Arlene and conducting some tests, we learned that although Arlene was eating reasonably well, she was not absorbing vitamin $B_{12}$, as well as several other nutrients, adequately. Arlene's physician had prescribed omeprazole (Prilosec) for gastroesophageal reflux disease (GERD), and this drug contributed to the poor $B_{12}$ absorption.

When Arlene and Ellie first walked into my office, they thought they were facing Alzheimer's disease; when they walked out, they had an intensive supplement and nutrition plan, including $B_{12}$ and folic acid injections over several weeks, which soon eliminated Arlene's symptoms. Arlene also spoke with her primary physician about stopping omeprazole.

Vitamin $B_{12}$ is involved in methylation (see the introduction to part 2), in which methyl $B_{12}$ helps to process homocysteine back to methionine. Other forms of supplemental $B_{12}$ (namely, cyanocobalamin and hydroxocobalamin) must be converted in the body to methyl $B_{12}$ or adenosyl $B_{12}$ to be used. Vitamin $B_{12}$ also works intimately with folic acid and essential fatty acids and is crucial in the development of the myelin sheath that insulates nerve fibers and allows for the free movement of neurotransmitters.

Although $B_{12}$ is absorbed into the body near the end of the small intestine (ileum), it requires a substance secreted in the stomach (intrinsic factor) to be properly absorbed. When this substance is absent, individuals develop pernicious anemia, a $B_{12}$ deficiency disease characterized by low numbers of large red blood cells and neurological and cognitive symptoms. People with dysbiosis (overgrowth of disease-causing bacteria or yeast in the gut) or with an inflamed ileum frequently do not properly absorb $B_{12}$.

Serum vitamin $B_{12}$ levels are not always a good reflection of how well the body is using $B_{12}$. A more sensitive test is the methylmalonic acid test, either from the blood or from the urine. $B_{12}$ is used to metabolize methylmalonic acid, and when it is high, this suggests a $B_{12}$ deficiency. Even this test is not sensitive enough, however, because if there is a problem making methyl $B_{12}$ or methylcobalamin (again, see the introduction to part 2), methylmalonic acid could be normal along with a $B_{12}$ deficiency. Sometimes serum levels of $B_{12}$ are very high, yet the individual still has a relative deficiency. Therefore, supplementation with methyl $B_{12}$ may be needed. For example, if the enzyme needed to convert homocysteine back to methionine is damaged by mercury or other toxins, high doses of methyl $B_{12}$ given by injection a few times a week may help the damaged enzyme to work better and improve methylation.

Elevated serum homocysteine levels may also occur as a result of vitamin $B_{12}$ (but also folic acid or vitamin $B_6$) deficiency. Fatigue and depression are two of the most common symptoms of mild $B_{12}$ deficiency. Sometimes treatment with either sublingual (under-the-tongue) $B_{12}$ tablets or injections can help to determine if there is a relative $B_{12}$ deficiency.

In addition to older adults, a vitamin $B_{12}$ deficiency is frequently seen among alcoholics and vegans (individuals who do not eat any foods derived from animals). Good food sources of vitamin $B_{12}$ include beef and chicken liver, clams, oysters, eggs, tempeh, sea vegetables, brewer's yeast, bee pollen, and mushrooms. Supplementation with vitamin $B_{12}$ can be by injection for people who are severely deficient, or by sublingual tablets, 500 mcg twice a day, for those with less serious deficiencies. An optimal maintenance dose is 50 to 100 mcg daily.

## Folic Acid

A deficiency of folic acid, or folate, is one of the most common vitamin deficiencies in the United States. Much of this is due to excessive alcohol intake (representing 5 percent of the US population) and pregnancy (20 percent of pregnant women have a folic acid deficiency because they have a much greater need for folate than nonpregnant women). At the same time, depression is one of the most common symptoms of a folic acid deficiency. A 2004 study of more than twenty-three hundred men who were followed for eleven to fifteen years showed that low levels of dietary folic acid may be a risk factor for severe depression. In addition, folic acid deficiency is associated with bipolar disorder, dementia, insomnia, irritability, and restless leg syndrome.

From our discussion of methylation, we know that folic acid donates a methyl group to vitamin $B_{12}$ to regenerate methionine and thus promotes methylation. Recall that methyl groups are critical for the synthesis of certain neurotransmitters, and a deficiency of folic acid has been linked with low levels of serotonin and S-adenosylmethionine (SAMe)—an amino acid metabolite that helps lift mood. Folic acid is also necessary to make dopamine, norepinephrine, and epinephrine.

Folic acid has even proved helpful in enhancing the efficacy of antidepressants. In a British study of 127 depressed individuals, researchers gave fluoxetine (Prozac) plus 500 mcg of folic acid to half of the patients and fluoxetine plus placebo to the other half. Among the women in the folic acid group, the addition of the vitamin significantly improved the antidepressant action of fluoxetine and minimized the drug's side effects. The same was not true, however, for the men who received the folic acid, who appear to require a higher dose of folic acid to achieve the same results.

The RDA for folic acid is 400 mcg per day, but if you are depressed, at least 800 mcg is recommended. Foods rich in folic acid include green leafy vegetables, whole wheat bread, and bananas, among others (see chapter 7). Because supplementation with folic acid can mask a vitamin $B_{12}$ deficiency, I recommend also taking a balanced B-complex vitamin that contains at least 300 mcg of vitamin $B_{12}$.

## CHOLINE

Choline isn't exactly a vitamin, since the body is capable of making it, but is a valuable accessory food factor associated with the vitamin B complex. Choline is often linked with inositol, another accessory food factor, and they often are found together in foods and in supplements. Choline is involved in the release and production of various neurotransmitters, but especially acetylcholine, which is associated with mood, memory, and alertness. European researchers found that injections of choline eliminated depression in patients who were suffering from depression, anxiety, sleeplessness, and paranoia. Choline may also improve mood in people who have Alzheimer's disease.

Individuals who benefit most from choline supplementation include those who have depression related to memory loss, lack of mental energy, or cognitive difficulties. A good natural source of choline is lecithin, an oily substance obtained from corn and soybeans that's available in granules, oil-filled capsules, and liquid form. Another form is phosphatidyl choline. The recommended daily dose is 1,000 to 2,000 mg of 90 percent pure phosphatidyl choline or 5 to 10 g of lecithin that is 20 percent phosphatidyl choline. Food sources include egg yolks, green leafy vegetables, wheat germ, liver, and peanuts.

Injectable phosphatidyl choline—along with injectable glutathione—has been used successfully at the Schachter Center to help depressed patients who are experiencing memory or other cognitive problems. This treatment, which has been successful in Europe, may be given from once a week to daily, depending upon the patient's condition. Several of my patients have improved significantly with this therapy.

## INOSITOL

In 1999, a rat study conducted in Israel showed that a nutrient called inositol, which the body can produce itself as well as obtain from both plant and animal sources, held great promise as a treatment for depression. Since then, its importance in treating mood disorders has been demonstrated in a few studies, including one in which 12 g of inositol was given to depressed patients in a double-blind, placebo-controlled study. After four weeks, the treatment group showed significant improvement compared with the placebo group. Other studies have produced similar results, with inositol also proving effective in reducing panic attacks and in treating obsessive-compulsive disorder.

At the Schachter Center, we frequently administer inositol in the dosages used in the Israeli studies. We recommend between a half (2.5 g) and a full teaspoonful (5 g) of inositol powder dissolved in a glass of water three times daily. We use this along with targeted amino acids, balanced fatty acids, and the various other methods described in this book. Our results have been excellent. It has also proved helpful in improving sleep problems.

Inositol appears to have a direct effect on neurotransmitters such as serotonin in the brain, and may be especially helpful if your depression is related to an anxiety disorder. Inositol is available in capsules, tablets, powder, and liquid. Food sources include bananas, wheat germ, citrus, cantaloupe, beans, nuts, whole grains, and brewer's yeast. The recommended maintenance dose of inositol for adults is 250 to 500 mg, while treatment doses are much higher, as noted above. However, use of this nutrient is safe and nontoxic, even at levels much greater than those recommended.

## VITAMIN A AND BETA-CAROTENE

Vitamin A, a fat-soluble nutrient, and beta-carotene (or pro-vitamin A, which can be converted in the body into vitamin A as needed) both play an indirect but important role in depression. For example, depression is often associated with stress or underlying medical conditions, such as premenstrual syndrome, fibromyalgia, or chronic fatigue syndrome, and vitamin A can help protect the body from the low mood and other symptoms associated with these conditions.

I often recommend about 5,000 International Units (IU) daily for adults, but may recommend much higher doses for brief periods. An RDA has not been established for beta-carotene, which I usually prescribe as part of a mixture of carotenes with dosage for adults being in the range of 25,000 IU (15 mg). A convenient way to take vitamin A, vitamin D, and omega-3 fatty acids is cod liver oil. Look for naturally flavored brands free of mercury and other toxins. I usually recommend between a teaspoonful and a tablespoonful a day. It is also available as gel capsules.

## VITAMIN C

The key point about vitamin C (ascorbic acid) is that most mammals are able to make it, but humans lost this ability and must ingest it from food or supplements. The late great Linus Pauling, PhD, popularized the notion of adding vitamin C to a supplement program. Many people associate vitamin C with an ability to fight colds or ward off flu symptoms, but this versatile vitamin also plays a significant role in the synthesis of dopamine and norepinephrine, is required for conversion of

5-HTP to serotonin, aids in the absorption of iron, helps strengthen the adrenals and several other glands, and is critical for the metabolism of essential fatty acids. The classic indication of a vitamin C deficiency is scurvy, which is rarely seen in the United States today. However, other symptoms of a vitamin C deficiency include depression and confusion (the earliest signs of a vitamin C deficiency), fatigue, apathy, and weakness.

You risk having low levels of vitamin C if you use oral contraceptives or tetracycline or if you are pregnant, elderly, or under a lot of stress. Supplementation with vitamin C may be beneficial if your depression is related to poor norepinephrine or dopamine activity, stress, an imbalance or deficiency of essential fatty acids, or the presence of a connective tissue condition. However, it is relatively easy to get a healthy amount of vitamin C from a diet that contains fruits and vegetables, especially citrus, peppers, strawberries, broccoli, kiwi, cauliflower, and turnip greens. The optimal therapeutic daily dose of vitamin C for adults is 500 to 3,000 mg. Supplementation is usually needed to reach these levels.

## VITAMIN D

When Dr. Michael Holick, a professor of medicine who heads the Vitamin D Laboratory at Boston University, was asked to step down as professor of dermatology at the same institution, it raised some eyebrows. What had this renowned expert on vitamin D done or said to cause this dismissal? He recommended that people spend some time in the sun, without sunscreen—a mere ten to fifteen minutes per day—so the body can make vitamin D. He noted that exposure to the sun's ultraviolet B rays supplies more than 90 percent of a person's vitamin D. Thus, insufficient sun exposure often results in a vitamin D deficiency. Dr. Holick may have been fired from his position because he criticized dermatologists who suggested that all sunlight exposure should be avoided because it causes cancer. Holick believes that a limited amount of bright sun exposure on skin without suntan lotion is necessary and desirable for optimal health.

Vitamin D isn't exactly a vitamin, because it can be made by the body from cholesterol in the skin when the skin is exposed to bright sunlight. The cholesterol converts to cholecalciferol, which travels to the liver, where it converts to 25-hydroxyvitamin D (not a very active form). This then travels to the kidneys, where the active form, 1,25-dihydroxyvitamin D, is made. The best way to assess a person's vitamin D status is to measure the serum 25-hydroxyvitamin D, a blood test.

While most people are aware that excessive sun exposure is a risk factor for some types of skin cancer and that vitamin D is necessary for strong bones, less well known are the connections among sunlight, vitamin D, and depression. Vitamin D in the adrenal glands regulates tyrosine hydroxylase, an enzyme that is necessary for the production of dopamine, epinephrine, and norepinephrine. Therefore, low levels of vitamin D can hinder the manufacture of these neurotransmitters and contribute to depression and fatigue.

I mentioned previously that the type of depression usually associated with insufficient sun exposure and vitamin D deficiency is seasonal affective disorder (SAD). A lack of sunlight disrupts the production of melatonin, a hormone that regulates the sleep–wake cycle, by the pineal gland. Less melatonin is released during the night, resulting in poor sleep quality and people waking up tired and depressed. Both light therapy (see chapter 10) and vitamin D are effective in the treatment of SAD, which affects about eleven million Americans.

In the 1980s, Professor Walter E. Stumpf of the University of North Carolina, a pioneer in vitamin D research, predicted a substantial role for both bright light and vitamin D in psychiatry. Although bright light can positively affect mood without creating vitamin D in the body, the vitamin also appears to improve mood as a supplement, independent of light. In a 1998 experiment, Australian researchers found that cholecalciferol (400 and 800 IU) significantly enhanced positive mood when given to healthy individuals. In 1999, scientists Bruce Hollis, Michael Gloth, and Wasif Alam found that 100,000 IU of vitamin D, given as a onetime oral dose, improved depression better than light therapy in a small group of patients with SAD.

How does vitamin D affect the brain? Summer sunlight increases brain serotonin levels twice as high as winter sunlight, which is compatible with both bright light in the visible spectrum and vitamin D affecting mood. Vitamin D also stimulates the production of norepinephrine.

A large percentage of the population is deficient in vitamin D, with 25-hydroxyvitamin D levels below 30 ng/ml (nanograms per milliliter). At the Schachter Center, we check all depressed patients for vitamin D deficiency and prescribe a supplement for anyone with levels less than 30 ng/ml. The optimal level is probably 45 to 60 ng/ml, and the dosage we recommend in most cases is 1,000 to 4,000 IU daily.

# VITAMIN E

One of the main functions of this fat-soluble vitamin is as an antioxidant—to protect the body, including the neurons in the brain, against the damaging effects of free radicals. Major depression is associated with defective antioxidant functioning, and so ensuring healthy antioxidant activity is important in the fight against depression. One recent study looked at vitamin E levels in patients with major depression and in healthy controls and found that levels in depressed individuals were significantly lower than those in the controls. Vitamin E can be helpful if your depression is related to stress, an underlying medical condition (especially heart disease), or inadequate serotonin activity.

Food sources of vitamin E include vegetable oils, including corn, wheat germ, and safflower, as well as dark green leafy vegetables, whole grains, nuts, seeds, and legumes. Vitamin E supplements can be either natural or synthetic. Natural (D-alpha tocopherol) is more bioavailable and better retained by the body than the more common synthetic form, DL-alpha tocopherol, and thus is two to three times more potent. Until recently, clinicians have focused on alpha tocopherol, but recent research indicates that gamma tocopherol may be at least as important and perhaps more important than alpha tocopherol for many conditions.

I strongly advise against the synthetic form of vitamin E, despite its lower price. Although much of the research has focused on D-alpha tocopherol, there are other forms of vitamin-E-related compounds, including beta, gamma, and delta tocopherols and alpha, beta, gamma, and delta tocotrienols. I recommend vitamin E supplements that contain at least all of the tocopherols (mixed tocopherols) and preferably one that also contains the tocotrienols. The optimal daily dose for adults is 200 to 800 IU. In some studies of neurological conditions, however, much higher dosages seem to be effective. Nevertheless, excessive daily use (1,200 IU or greater) may cause elevated blood pressure, dizziness, or decreased blood coagulation in some patients.

## CALCIUM AND MAGNESIUM

We consider calcium and magnesium together because these minerals work in sync. Both are essential for healthy functioning of the central nervous system and are often regarded as the body's natural tranquilizers. In particular, calcium is necessary for proper serotonin function, as well as prevention of depression and irritability. In two double-blind, placebo-controlled studies of college-aged subjects, for example, researchers found that supplementation with calcium (1,000 mg plus 600 mg vitamin D, twice daily) resulted in a significant improvement in mood when compared with controls.

Magnesium helps maintain blood sugar balance; when levels are low, it is associated with depression, anxiety, irritability, and fatigue. Anyone familiar with premenstrual syndrome will recognize these symptoms. Supplementation with magnesium alleviates these very symptoms, and thus is helpful to many people suffering with depression.

I find that magnesium is particularly beneficial for patients suffering from anxiety and heart palpitations. Several magnesium supplements are well absorbed, including magnesium glycinate, citrate, and amino acid chelate. My favorite for most patients is magnesium taurate, which is a combination of magnesium and taurine. These substances enhance each other, reducing anxiety and cardiac arrhythmias. For some people, magnesium may cause loose stools; I treat this by lowering the dose.

Of the many available calcium supplements, calcium carbonate contains a greater amount of calcium than, say, calcium citrate, which is better absorbed but requires taking more pills (the amount of calcium per pill is less than that for carbonate). Calcium causes constipation in some people.

Supplementation with calcium and magnesium may be especially helpful if your depression is related to an imbalance in blood sugar or to an imbalance or deficiency in essential fatty acids. Calcium citrate also stimulates cellular processes that cause the release of epinephrine. The recommended daily dose of calcium is 500 mg to 1,500 mg, which should be balanced with intake of roughly between half and an equal amount of magnesium. There is some controversy about whether calcium and magnesium should be taken in the same capsule or separately, because there is evidence that they may interfere with each other's absorption. I usually decide on an individual basis. If, for example, I think it is important for the patient to take magnesium taurate, I give this separately from calcium. Most people think of dairy foods when calcium is mentioned, but dark green leafy vegetables such as kale and collards are very good sources, as are sesame seeds, nuts, and beans. Food sources of magnesium include whole grains, nuts, seeds, green leafy vegetables, tofu, legumes, avocados, and many fruits and vegetables.

## CHROMIUM

Chromium is a mineral that forms part of a compound known as glucose tolerance factor, which helps keep blood sugar (glucose) levels in balance by enhancing the effects of insulin. Low levels of chromium reduce the effectiveness of insulin and can lead to glucose intolerance. The body does not absorb chromium efficiently, so it is often combined with an amino acid derivative (such as picolinic acid, a derivative of tryptophan, to form chromium picolinate) or a vitamin (say, niacin in polynicotinate) to improve absorption.

Research showing a positive impact of chromium on depressive symptoms has not been around long, but it is convincing. In 1999, University of North Carolina psychiatrists found that supplementation with 200 to 400 mcg of chromium picolinate per day in patients with dysthymic mood disorder caused rapid "mood-elevating effects," which they attributed to the mineral's ability to boost the body's use of glucose and, possibly, its ability to enhance neurotransmitter activity in the brain.

Subsequently, in a placebo-controlled, double-blind study conducted at Duke University Medical Center, 70 percent of patients with major depressive disorder who were given 600 mcg of chromium picolinate for eight weeks improved, while none of the patients on placebo did. Researchers speculate that the promising results may be related to the effect of chromium on serotonin receptors, increased sensitivity to insulin, or other reasons.

In another study, eight depressed patients who had not responded to other treatments were given chromium supplements, to which they responded with a "dramatic" improvement in their symptoms, again related to its positive effect on insulin utilization. At the same time, chromium use was associated with an increase in the availability of tryptophan.

At the Schachter Center, most patients are checked for chromium and other mineral status with a red blood cell mineral analysis. Low levels are treated with supplementation. Additional chromium in the diet is encouraged as well, but chromium is present in only low levels in most foods, with the best sources being whole grains, brewer's yeast, potatoes, and wheat germ. No daily recommended allowance has been established for chromium, but the estimated safe and adequate daily dietary intake is 50 to 200 mcg. If you have bipolar disorder, chromium should be used with caution, because any nutrient or medication that improves depression may potentially trigger a hypomanic or manic episode in some individuals. Similarly, if you have diabetes and are taking insulin or any type of diabetes medication, first talk with your health-care practitioner. Chromium supplementation can decrease insulin resistance and thus have an impact on the amount of medication you may need to take.

## IRON

When we think of iron deficiency, anemia is usually the first thing that comes to mind. However, iron deficiency anemia is generally a late manifestation of this condition. Symptoms of fatigue and exhaustion from iron deficiency may show up before the anemia appears and can be treated with iron supplementation.

Iron deficiency also has an impact on neurotransmitter production, because it is involved in the synthesis of serotonin, norepinephrine, and dopamine. Thus the low mood associated with iron deficiency is associated with a neurotransmitter imbalance. An iron deficiency may also cause an imbalance in nutrients that are important in mood, including zinc and copper, as well as contributing to hypothyroidism, which is associated with depression (see chapter 9): Iron is instrumental in the conversion of phenylalanine to tyrosine, a precursor of thyroid hormones.

Iron is readily stored in the body, and an excessive accumulation can contribute to serious medical problems, including cardiovascular disease. Therefore, do not take an iron supplement or a multinutrient that contains iron unless an iron deficiency is present. The optimal daily dose of iron for an adult is 15 to 20 mg, or more if there is a deficiency, but no iron supplement is necessary if there is not.

At the Schachter Center, virtually every patient has a serum ferritin test to determine iron levels (see chapter 3). Ferritin is a protein found in the body that binds iron. Normal laboratory ranges are usually much too wide and do not consider the damaging effects of moderately elevated iron. We generally like to see the ferritin somewhere between 30 and 80. Good food sources of iron include raisins, almonds, cashews, wheat germ, brewer's yeast, sesame seeds, whole grains, legumes, meat, and dark green leafy vegetables.

## POTASSIUM

Potassium is a mineral that plays an essential role in maintaining proper functioning of nervous system tissues and cell growth. A deficiency may cause depression, severe weakness and fatigue, nervousness, headache, and irregular heartbeat.

A potassium deficiency may be more common than many people think, largely because it can be caused by consuming high-salt foods, processed foods, and lots of alcohol or caffeine, common habits in the United States. It can also be caused by stress. The adrenal glands respond to stress by secreting increased levels of steroid hormones in the brain, causing the kidneys to reabsorb sodium and lose potassium into the urine, depleting potassium levels. Another major cause of potassium deficiency is diuretics (water pills), which are used extensively to treat high blood pressure and congestive heart failure. Frequently, magnesium deficiency and potassium deficiency occur together, because the same factors cause both conditions—a fact often not recognized by physicians. It is very difficult for the body to hold on to potassium if there is a magnesium deficiency, and both should be corrected simultaneously.

Potassium is found primarily within cells rather than in the bloodstream, therefore serum blood levels of potassium are not very good for detecting subtle deficiencies. You can lose 50 percent of body potassium and still have a normal serum potassium. When serum potassium is low, this means that the body is quite deficient in potassium. Although no official daily allowance of potassium has been named, experts largely agree that 2,000 to 3,500 mg per day is healthy. Good food sources include apricots, apples, oranges and grapefruits and their juices, bananas, broccoli, leafy green vegetables, peas, potatoes, and tomatoes. Potassium supplements are available in dosages up to 99 mg per tablet or capsule; higher doses (for instance, 600 mg per tablet or capsule) are available by prescription.

## SELENIUM

Several studies indicate that low levels of the mineral selenium are associated with depressed mood, and that depressed individuals who have low levels of selenium experience an improvement in mood after taking supplements or eating a high-selenium diet. In one study, fifty people were given either 100 mcg of selenium or a placebo over five weeks. Participants monitored their mood and feelings during the study and reported on the foods they ate as well. At the end of the study, the researchers found that the lower the level of selenium in the diet, the more the individuals reported feelings of depression, anxiety, and fatigue. They also found that these feelings disappeared when selenium supplements were added to the diet.

Selenium also plays a role in mood in another way: It is necessary for optimal synthesis and metabolism of thyroid hormone, and thyroid function affects mood and behavior. Thus it's important to get an optimal amount of selenium from foods such as Brazil nuts, brewer's yeast, fish, garlic, grains, shellfish, and sunflower seeds, or from a supplement. The optimal daily dose is 100 to 200 mcg. Excessive amounts (more than 3,200 mcg daily) can cause neurological abnormalities, hair loss, and paralysis. Selenium status can be checked by the red blood cell mineral test.

## ZINC AND COPPER

We're looking at zinc and copper together because zinc affects copper levels and vice versa. It is important to maintain a proper ratio between these two minerals. When supplementing, a good ratio of zinc to copper is about 7:1 or 14:1. Individually, however, they have different functions when it comes to depression. Zinc is a cofactor for many different enzymes, including some involved in the synthesis of serotonin, norepinephrine, and GABA. It also promotes the development of brain cells and is necessary for maintaining an optimal balance of estrogen, progesterone, and testosterone, discussed in chapter 9. Zinc is also required for metabolism of thyroid-stimulating hormone (TSH), which is necessary for healthy thyroid function.

Copper is necessary for the synthesis of norepinephrine and thus helps maintain an optimal norepinephrine-to-dopamine ratio. It is also involved in the synthesis of myelin, the coating that insulates nerve fibers, and is a cofactor for the enzyme monoamine oxidase, which helps in the degradation of serotonin, norepinephrine, dopamine, and epinephrine. So copper deficiency can contribute to depression, but an excess can also cause depression, as well as mood swings, headache, fatigue, memory problems, and hyperactivity.

Dietary sources of zinc include pumpkin seeds, oysters, organ meats, dairy products, lentils, beans, and whole grains. Copper is plentiful in shellfish, liver, dark green leafy vegetables, nuts, mushrooms, and dried fruit. The recommended daily allowance for adults for copper is 2 mg; for zinc, 12 mg for females and 15 mg for males, but therapeutic doses can be higher for limited periods of time.

## IODINE

My thinking about iodine is undergoing a major transition as I write this book, thanks to the work of Guy Abraham, MD, former professor of obstetrics, gynecology, and endocrinology at the UCLA School of Medicine. Through his series of articles, termed *The Iodine Project*, Dr. Abraham has suggested that the optimal daily dose of iodine is approximately 12.5 mg, which is one hundred times the RDA of 0.125 mg. He believes that the current prevailing medical opinion that more than 2 mg a day of iodine is toxic is wrong, and he traces the source of this major blunder to a 1948 scientific experiment on rats that was later generalized to humans.

Although it has long been believed that iodine's only role in the body is to help make thyroid hormones, Abraham describes other functions, including but not limited to helping to regulate mood and preventing cancer (especially in breasts, ovaries, uterus, prostate, and thyroid gland). For example, Japanese women, who have one of the lowest breast cancer rates in the world, ingest more than 13 mg of iodine daily from seaweed and do not seem to suffer any adverse consequences. He further shows that iodine tends to be antibacterial, antiviral, antiparasitic, and antifungal; that it enhances immune function; and that insufficient iodine intake may contribute to various common thyroid abnormalities, including hypothyroidism, hyperthyroidism, and autoimmune inflammation of the thyroid (Hashimoto's disease). These conditions are all worsened when a person is exposed to substances that damage the thyroid gland, such as bromide and fluoride.

In the 1820s, the French physician Jean Lugol combined elemental iodine (5 percent) and potassium iodide (10 percent) with 85 percent water. Since iodine kills infectious agents, Dr. Lugol successfully treated many infectious conditions with this solution, which was named Lugol's solution and is still available today by prescription.

In his excellent book on iodine, *Iodine: Why You Need It, Why You Can't Live Without It*, Dr. David Brownstein summarized his experience with hundreds of patients for whom he has prescribed iodine with excellent results and minimal side effects. To determine whether patients are iodine-sufficient, he uses the iodine-loading test described by Dr. Abraham and now in use at the Schachter Center. Patients empty their bladder and ingest 50 mg of iodine/iodide (discussed further below). They then collect their urine for the next twenty-four hours and send a sample of it along with a note that includes the total volume to an appropriate laboratory. People who excrete 90 percent or 45 mg of the iodine are iodine-sufficient. A therapeutic dosage of iodine is given for a period of time if less than 45 mg is excreted. A few months later the person is retested. Using this test, Dr. Brownstein has found that more than 90 percent of his patients are iodine-insufficient before iodine treatment is begun.

Once a person is iodine-sufficient, the maintenance dose for an adult to maintain sufficiency is about 12.5 mg of iodine/iodide daily according to Dr. Brownstein, and this can be obtained with two drops of Lugol's solution. This high dose of iodine may have other benefits as well, as Dr. Abraham has shown that iodine promotes the excretion of toxic minerals such as lead, mercury, and cadmium as well as fluoride and bromide. In the May 2005 edition of *Nutrition and Healing*, Dr. Jonathan V. Wright noted that his laboratory has also shown that iodine helps remove toxic elements. When toxins are mobilized, patients may develop side effects such as fatigue and irritability, which can be reduced by lowering the dosage of iodine and making sure that other aspects of nutrition and nutritional supplementation are in place. A physician knowledgeable about iodine who can order tests when necessary should monitor all of this.

Although our experience at the Schachter Center with iodine is limited as of this writing, I believe its use offers help to patients with depression and many other symptoms, especially those associated with the thyroid gland. One patient whom I've been following for episodes of depression for a few years had developed significant hair loss for several months, which was unresponsive to thyroid hormone supplementation, biotin, extra protein, and other measures that I usually recommend for hair loss. On 37.5 mg of iodine for six weeks, this condition completely cleared; the treatment also helped to stabilize her mood.

On the other hand, we've had some patients develop side effects, such as the worsening of low thyroid symptoms and an elevation of TSH (indicating low thyroid function) with dosages of iodine/iodide as low as 12.5 mg and suspect problems may occur even at 6 mg daily for some people. This may be caused by the iodine mobilizing thyroid-damaging substances, such as bromide and fluoride from the tissues, resulting in an adverse effect on thyroid functioning. Patients taking dosages of more than 5 mg per day of iodine/iodide should be watched closely by a practitioner familiar with its use. I generally have been starting patients at dosages of about 5 mg of iodine/iodide daily and raise the dosage slowly and carefully, if at all, cautioning patients about possible adverse effects.

Currently, iodine deficiency is considered in all depressed patients at the Schachter Center.

## CONCENTRATED FRUIT AND VEGETABLE EXTRACTS

Although I firmly believe the ideal way for people to get their nutrients is from organic whole foods, it is often necessary to enhance even the best diet with supplements, especially when treating a medical condition. For some of my patients, the optimal way to provide them with the nutrients they need has been through use of concentrated nutraceuticals—supplements that have nutritional and/or therapeutic value for maintaining health or treating disease. Specifically, I am talking about an extract of many different fruits and/or vegetables in one convenient capsule. Typically, these supplements begin as fruits and/or vegetables that are processed to extract their phytonutrients (active chemicals such as bioflavonoids, carotenoids, polyphenols, and others), removing water, sugar, salt, and fiber, and reducing what remains to a capsule or tablet. Removal of the fiber improves absorption of these supplements, while elimination of sugars makes them suitable for people who have *Candida* or blood sugar problems.

What's so special about these concentrated nutraceuticals? Unlike most vitamin and mineral supplements, they are made from whole fresh foods. Most traditional supplements, however, are synthesized from coal tar, petroleum chemicals, mineral ores, shells, and animal by-products. In many cases, fillers such as soy, lactose, starch, and magnesium sulfate are added as well.

Concentrated fruit and vegetable nutraceuticals are made by several different companies (see the appendix), each with its own special formula.

## HERBAL REMEDIES

The addition of herbal remedies to a depression treatment program can be very rewarding, especially for individuals who suffer with mild to moderate depression. Indeed, such therapies have been broadly used throughout Europe for decades. Generally, the benefits of these remedies come on more gradually than those associated with medications, but their side effects are minimal or nonexistent. This feature makes them especially attractive to people who have experienced adverse reactions, such as agitation, sexual dysfunction, dry mouth, and weight gain, when using prescription antidepressants.

Here I examine four herbal remedies: St.-John's-wort, ginseng, *Ginkgo biloba*, and rhodiola. St.-John's-wort has had much press in recent years, some good and some not so favorable. Ginseng and ginkgo have been the subjects of increasing scrutiny in the area of depression, while rhodiola is a relative newcomer that has much promise.

### St.-John's-Wort

St.-John's-wort (*Hypericum perforatum*) is a plant that contains many chemical compounds, including hypericin and hyperforin, that may be helpful in the treatment of mild to moderate depression for some individuals, especially those who have a serotonin deficiency and/or who are experiencing anxiety and sleep disturbances. St.-John's-wort works by inhibiting an enzyme (catechol-O-methyltransferase) that degrades some neurotransmitters, including dopamine. This herb also mimics the actions of selective serotonin reuptake inhibitors (see chapter 12)—it, too, inhibits serotonin reuptake in the brain.

These actions help relieve depression by slowing the recycling of neurotransmitters that the brain needs to maintain emotional balance.

Reports of the effectiveness of St.-John's-wort in the treatment of depression are mixed. A review of twenty-three randomized trials (totaling 1,757 participants) looked at fifteen placebo-controlled studies and eight that compared the herb with an antidepressant. St.-John's-wort was nearly three times more effective than placebo and comparable in effect to prescription antidepressants, including imipramine, diazepam, and amitriptyline, but with fewer and less severe side effects. In fact, 52.8 percent of patients who took prescription antidepressants experienced side effects compared with only 19.8 percent of those taking St.-John's-wort.

In a more recent study (*British Medical Journal*, February 2005), an extract of St.-John's-wort was compared with paroxetine (Paxil) in more than 250 people who had moderate to severe depression. The results of the double-blind, placebo-controlled study showed that after six weeks of treatment, the extract was at least as effective as the drug, and was better tolerated.

Other reports, however, are not as promising. In a double-blind trial that involved 340 participants, St.-John's-wort was no more effective for treating major depression than placebo. However, this study also found that sertraline (Zoloft), an SSRI medication, was no better than placebo on the main measures of depression, although it did fare better than placebo on one clinical scale.

If you use St.-John's-wort, keep a few caveats in mind. Because of potential herb–drug interactions, do not use this herb along with MAOIs such as Nardil or Parnate, or with SSRIs like Prozac, Zoloft, and Celexa. In addition, use of St.-John's-wort reduces the effectiveness of many drugs, including but not limited to amitriptyline, cyclosporine, digoxin, oral contraceptives, theophylline, warfarin, and some anticancer drugs. In addition, St.-John's-wort can, on rare occasions, aggravate mania, so it must be used with caution and under medical supervision if you have a bipolar condition. Given these possible interactions, it is important to work with a knowledgeable health-care practitioner when using St.-John's-wort.

### Ginkgo Biloba

In both Europe and the United States, *Ginkgo biloba* is one of the most widely used natural remedies to boost mood and improve memory. Research shows that ginkgo stimulates blood circulation throughout the body, including the brain, which helps reverse short-term memory loss and relieve depression and lethargy. It also helps protect nerve cells in the brain from free radical damage. The compounds believed to be responsible for ginkgo's positive effects include flavoglycosides and terpene lactones.

In the treatment of depression, ginkgo shows the most promise among adults fifty and older. In one study, elderly depressed patients who had not responded to antidepressant therapy did respond when *Ginkgo biloba* was added to their treatment regimen. Experts speculate that ginkgo helps relieve depression by increasing the numbers of serotonin binding sites in the brain, which normally decrease with age.

The most widely used ginkgo products are extracts standardized to 24 percent of flavoglycosides and 6 percent terpene lactones. For adults, the usual daily dose of a standardized extract is 40 mg three times a day, though higher doses have been used.

Because *Ginkgo biloba* increases blood circulation, it may cause bleeding if used by anyone who is also taking blood-thinning agents, such as aspirin or warfarin. If you are taking such drugs or if you have a history of hemorrhaging, do not use this herb.

## Siberian Ginseng

An interesting fact about Siberian ginseng (*Eleutherococcus senticosus*) is that it is not true ginseng, even though it is in the same family as American and Chinese ginseng. Thus, it has different characteristics than its cousins. In addition, Siberian ginseng is an *adaptogen*—an agent that strengthens the body and helps it return to normal after stressful episodes. Apparently, Siberian ginseng has this ability because it contains substances that have a positive effect on the adrenal glands and that fight the symptoms of stress, such as insomnia, fatigue, and mood swings. These abilities help make Siberian ginseng a good choice if your depression is related to stress or to the presence of a chronic illness.

The recommended daily dose of Siberian ginseng for adults is 200 mg of an extract standardized for 1 percent eleutherosides. Siberian ginseng may cause restlessness and nervousness in some people and insomnia if taken close to bedtime. This herb should be used cautiously under medical supervision if high blood pressure is present. If you experience tightness in your chest or throat, breathing problems, chest pain, itchy skin, or a rash, this may be due to Siberian ginseng, which should be discontinued. This herb may interact with some prescription drugs, including heart medications, stimulants, barbiturates, diabetic medicine (including insulin and glipizide), and antipsychotic drugs. If you are taking these or any other medications, talk to your health-care practitioner before starting supplementation with ginseng.

## Rhodiola

Rhodiola is an herb that has long been used in Russia and Scandinavia to relieve depression, boost energy, eliminate fatigue, and prevent altitude sickness. Like Siberian ginseng, rhodiola is classified as an adaptogen because of its ability to increase resistance to various stressors. Although I have no personal experience with rhodiola, recent research, much of which has been done in Russia and Europe, suggests that its adaptogenic activities may be due to its ability to influence endorphins and certain neurotransmitters and hormones, including serotonin, melatonin, and dopamine. Scientists report that unlike Siberian ginseng, which you need to take for several weeks before noting any benefit, rhodiola usually offers noticeable results after just one dose.

In a recent double-blind, placebo-controlled clinical study conducted in Russia, for example, 161 volunteers were given either one of two different doses of rhodiola or a placebo and then evaluated for the effect these substances had on their ability to perform mental work while fatigued and under stress. Individuals who were given rhodiola did significantly better than those who took a placebo.

Different studies of rhodiola have used various dosages; however, the suggested daily dose to treat chronic stress is 200 mg of extract standardized to 2 percent rosavins. Some studies have used as much as 200 mg taken two to three times daily.

## THE BOTTOM LINE

Supplementation with nutrients is a cornerstone of the ortho-molecular or functional medicine approach to treatment of depression. Planned supplementation, along with a healthful diet—discussed in the next chapter—can quickly put you back on the road to good mental health.

For an overview of the frequently used therapeutic doses of the nutrients discussed in this chapter, see the summary on page 174. Remember, these are approximate doses only; treatment doses may be greater, and any therapeutic program should be individualized to your specific biochemistry. Successful programs are frequently developed with the help of a nutritionally oriented health practitioner, but many people are able to develop effective programs by reading books such as this one and doing their own research. If you attempt a program on your own and develop any problems, seek help from a qualified health-care practitioner. Various resources, including organizations for nutritionally oriented practitioners, are found in the appendix.

# Optimal Doses of Nutrients That Help Relieve Depression

| Nutrient | Dose |
|---|---|
| B vitamins | |
|    Thiamine (vitamin $B_1$) | 10–100 mg |
|    Riboflavin (vitamin $B_2$) | 10–100 mg |
|    Niacin or niacinamide (vitamin $B_3$) | 10–1,000 mg |
|    Pantothenic acid (vitamin $B_5$) | 25–250 mg |
|    Pyridoxine (vitamin $B_6$) | 10–100 mg |
|    Folic acid | 400–1,200 mcg |
|    Vitamin $B_{12}$ | 50–1,000 mcg |
| Calcium | 500–1,500 mg |
| Choline | 250–2,000 mg |
| Chromium | 200–400 mcg |
| Copper | 1–2 mg |
| Inositol | 250–3,000 mg |
| Iodine/Iodide | 1–50 mg (with caution above 5 mg) |
| Iron | 0–6 mg (depending on iron sufficiency, usually reflected by serum ferritin) |
| Magnesium | 200–800 mg |
| NADH | 5–10 mg |
| Selenium | 50–200 mcg |
| Vitamin A | 2,500–10,000 IU |
| Vitamin C | 500–3,000 mg |
| Vitamin D | 800–10,000 IU |
| Vitamin E | 200–800 IU |
| Zinc | 12–15 mg |

## Chapter 7

## Eat Your Way Out of Depression

The promising news I want to share in this chapter is that you can make changes to your diet that will help you eat your way out of depression. The other news is that there is no one dietary formula for alleviating depression that works for everyone. When it comes to diet, one size does not fit all. This is true whether you want to lose weight or eat for better emotional and mental health, because each person has a unique biochemical makeup and specific nutritional needs that should be considered when choosing an optimal eating plan.

At the same time, there are certain basic nutritional guidelines that are essential for optimal emotional and mental health. Once you understand the foundation, your specific requirements can be met by making modifications to the basic plan.

In this chapter, I'll show you how you can choose the best foods to help combat depression. I begin with two lists—"Positive Foods" and "Foods to Avoid"—and explain the benefits and negative aspects of the items in each. I then discuss how you can optimize your diet and create your own healthy eating plan, which will address your unique nutritional needs, based on information from your checklists and, if you have them, test results from your health-care practitioner. Such a plan will include foods that provide a balance of amino acids, essential fatty acids, and nutrients discussed in previous chapters.

## IDENTIFYING A HEALTHFUL DIET

I admit it: It's hard to know what constitutes a healthful diet. It seems as if there's no end to the claims made by "experts" as to what you should be consuming: more fish or less fish, lots of milk or no milk, high-carb versus low-carb, high-protein versus low-protein, organic versus conventional, caffeine is okay or it's not okay.

Stephen, a thirty-four-year-old stockbroker, considered himself health-conscious. He watched his weight, played tennis a few times a week, and didn't smoke. But when he came to my office, he did not exude vitality: instead, he was depressed, shaky, and nervous. During his initial intake interview and examination, I ordered a red blood cell and mineral test, as I do with virtually all individuals who come to see me, and he talked with our nutritionist. That's when we learned that Stephen had fully embraced the idea that eating fish is healthy, so he was eating it five or six days a week. His intention to "eat healthy" was good, but his execution was not. His test results revealed that his body had accumulated mercury from his "healthy" diet, and he had the symptoms to prove it.

We told Stephen to immediately stop eating fish for the time being, and I started him on an oral chelation program (using the chelator dimercaptosuccinic acid, or DMSA) to help rid his body of mercury and other toxic minerals. Stephen worked with the nutritionist and developed a balanced eating plan that fit his needs, which eventually included a small amount of fish, and stressed whole organic grains, fruits, vegetables, and small amounts of organic lean meat. Within a few months, Stephen was feeling 100 percent better, and his red blood cell mercury returned to normal. His depression had lifted, and he boasted that his tennis game had greatly improved as well.

## Basics of a Healthful, Antidepression Diet

For some people, the phrase *healthful diet* is enough to send their mood tumbling. "Guess I'll have to give up everything I enjoy, like chocolate and hamburgers and french fries," sighed one patient. "That's enough to make me even more depressed!" But healthful need not be equated with unappetizing or boring. Different, perhaps, and for some people a change to a more healthful diet requires big adjustments—in the foods they buy, where they eat out, and how they prepare their choices. The rewards, however, are many, including improved mood, more energy, enhanced immune system, better concentration, and invigorated sex drive, to name but a few.

I've found that laying down a few basic but critical guidelines for a healthful diet, and then tweaking them for individual patients, works much better than expecting people to follow a complicated program that involves counting grams of carbohydrates or protein, weighing foods, referring to charts, or combining certain items in complicated ratios. That being said, here are my lists of "Positive Foods" and "Foods to Avoid."

## POSITIVE FOODS

• **Sweets.** In moderation, natural sugars such as rice syrup, date sugar, pure Vermont syrup, unsulfured blackstrap molasses, and unfiltered honey are all acceptable. An herbal sweetener—that has nearly no calories—is stevia, which can be found in health food stores and increasingly in mainstream grocery stores.

• **Fats.** As discussed in chapter 5, some fats are healthy and instrumental in maintaining mental health, especially omega-3 fatty acids. When you choose oil for cooking, your best choice is probably cold-pressed olive oil. Butter and other saturated fats (like coconut oil, but not margarine that contains trans-fatty acids) may be used in moderate amounts. I suggest you avoid fried foods (especially deep-fried).

• **Whole fruits and vegetables.** Whenever possible, choose fresh, organic fruits and vegetables and eat at least five to seven servings daily. To derive the most benefit from these rich sources of vitamins, minerals, fiber, and carbohydrates, eat them in as pure a state as possible, preferably raw or lightly steamed. (Sorry, deep-fried potatoes and onion rings don't count as servings of whole vegetables.) Fruit and vegetable juices are good as well, and if you have a juicer, please learn how to make your own fresh juices, remembering to drink the pulp as well!

• **Whole grains and cereals.** Whole grains and cereals (organic if possible) are excellent sources of complex carbohydrates. These foods include whole grains, brown rice, and unprocessed cereals. Complex carbohydrates break down gradually and provide a more steady supply of glucose—brain fuel—thus helping maintain an even or calmer mood. Simple carbohydrates, however, such as those found in sugary foods or those made with white flour, metabolize rapidly, contributing to and causing mood swings and energy highs and lows. Also, be aware that some grains and even other whole-food starches may be problematic for some people, as I explain on pages 189 to 193.

• **Beans, legumes, nuts, and seeds.** Choose organic foods in this important category as well. Foods in this group are excellent sources of protein, especially for people who want to reduce or eliminate animal protein. Beans, legumes, nuts, and seeds are also high in fiber and many nutrients. Also in this category are tofu and other forms of fermented soybeans (miso, tempeh) and flaxseed.

• **Eggs and dairy.** Eggs and dairy foods—milk, cheese, butter, cream, and yogurt—are good sources of protein, calcium, and other important nutrients. They are also rich sources of saturated fat, which may be fine for many people. The major concern I have about eggs and dairy relates to whether hormones were used in raising the animals; whether or not they were given foods containing pesticides, antibiotics, toxic minerals, or other chemicals; and whether the animals were confined to inhumane cages. Soft-boiled eggs are best because heat is applied without exposure to oxygen, thus reducing free radical damage. I recommend organic eggs and dairy products and prefer nonhomogenized milk. Although pasteurization of milk products is the norm today in order to eliminate harmful bacteria, certified raw milk is preferred in areas where it is available, provided the cows are clean and hygienic principles are used in caring for them. If you are lactose-intolerant because of a deficiency of the enzyme lactase, or you choose not to consume dairy items, nondairy foods may be used. These include products made from soy, rice, or nuts, such as soy milk, rice milk, and almond milk; cheese made from these "milks"; and nondairy desserts. These "dairy" foods are also good sources of protein.

• **Organic meats and poultry.** Despite a push for people to eat more fish, meat and poultry continue to be major sources of animal protein for many people. For patients who eat meat, I recommend organically raised products, which are virtually free of hormones, pesticides, antibiotics, and other unnatural additives, all of which can have a detrimental effect on mood and general health. Such meat and poultry choices are slowly becoming more accessible and typically are available in natural and whole-food stores. Meats and poultry are sources of methionine, which is critical for methylation (see the introduction to part 2); this amino acid is difficult to get from plant-based sources.

• **Fish and shellfish.** Fish and shellfish can be excellent sources of protein and omega-3 fatty acids, if you make judicious choices. I'm calling for "judicious choices" because of the persistent and very real problem of mercury, pesticides, PCBs, and other contamination of the fish supply. Fish that I tend to recommend that are high in omega-3 fatty acids, but relatively low in mercury, are wild Alaskan salmon and sardines. I am wary about farm-raised fish because some studies indicate that they are high in PCBs and other contaminants. The smaller the fish (say, sardines), the less likely they are to accumulate mercury. But if you eat fish fairly frequently, I recommend that you have your blood mercury levels checked, because there is no way to guarantee the fish you eat regularly is not contaminated. Everyone whom I have checked for mercury who eats sushi more than once a week is quite high in it. Swordfish, king mackerel, shark, and most tuna tend to be quite high in mercury.

I would like you to consider two factors when choosing foods from this list. One, do you have any reactions to these foods that may be contributing to or causing your depression? (See chapter 1 for discussion of food reactions.) Two, do you have any specific food preferences based on religious, ethical, and/or moral beliefs? If you are a vegetarian, for example, you will not select meat, poultry, or fish, so you will need to choose other protein-rich foods such as soy products, legumes, beans, seeds, and, depending on the type of vegetarian diet you follow, eggs and/or dairy.

### FOODS TO AVOID

Most of the foods included in this list should come as no surprise to you. In most cases, foods on the "Avoid" list have been highly refined and processed. Fortunately, for every food you should avoid, there is a healthy alternative on the "Positive Foods" list. You may find that the "Avoid" list reads like your current grocery list; or you may discover that only one or two categories apply to you. Next time you're in the grocery store, here are the items you want to skip:

• **Sugar.** Avoid all foods that contain added sugar, such as soda, candy, cakes, ketchup, some breakfast cereals, and so on. Become a label reader. If sugar (or one of its companions, such as corn syrup) is one of the first few ingredients, put the item back on the shelf! Sugar can give you a burst of energy, but in the long run it can leave you depressed and tired.

• **White-flour products.** Just say no to white bread, white pasta, and other products that use white flour, including many crackers, rolls and bagels, refrigerator biscuits, pizza dough, and baked goods. Also avoid white rice. These overly processed food products have been stripped of their nutritional value, and then they are "enriched" with some nutrients, along with synthetic additives.

• **Alcohol.** This includes beer, wine, and liquor. People often forget that alcohol is a depressant, even though it provides an initial kick. Drinking alcohol can also disturb your sleep, which is a problem with many people who are depressed.

• **Caffeine.** Avoid coffee, tea, colas, and chocolate. (Okay, you can have a *limited* amount of organic dark chocolate on occasion.) If you must have coffee, choose an organic coffee, since most coffees are high in pesticides. Decaffeinated coffee is fine for most people, provided that it is organic and does not use toxic chemicals in processing.

• **Hydrogenated fats.** Hydrogenated fats are oils to which hydrogen atoms have been added in the factory in order to harden them and improve shelf life (see chapter 5). These hydrogenated oils or fats contain high concentrations of trans-fatty acids, which have recently been clearly shown to disrupt fatty acid metabolism in the body and cause serious disease. Hydrogenated fats are found primarily in margarines, snack foods (potato chips, corn chips), crackers and cookies, baked products, and fast foods. When you read ingredient labels, look for the words *hydrogenated*, *partially hydrogenated*, *margarine*, or *shortening*, which indicate the presence of trans-fatty acids, or look at the nutritional panel for the percentage of trans-fat in the product. Beginning January 2006, food manufacturers were required to list trans-fat content on labels.

• **Chemical food additives.** To avoid artificial preservatives, flavorings, colors, and sweeteners, you need to read labels. Not all labels list all the chemicals in the food item, but the general rule is: If the product has been processed, it probably contains chemicals. For example, artificial preservatives such as BHA, BHT, nitrites, monosodium glutamate, and nitrates are often seen in cereals, breads, frozen dinners, boxed meals, and crackers. All foods containing artificial colors (such as red dye 40) or artificial flavorings should be avoided. Artificial additives can cause various adverse reactions, including mood swings, depression, fatigue, headache, rash, aggression, irritability, and attention difficulties, among others. I believe all artificial sweeteners, including saccharine, aspartame, and sucralose, should be avoided. In particular, avoid diet sodas containing aspartame.

• **Fluoride.** Do not drink fluoridated water or tap water (unless filtered) or use fluoridated toothpaste. Despite the popularity of fluoride dental treatments for both adults and children, I strongly recommend you not get them. Also, avoid fluoridated vitamins for children. There are a number of excellent books and websites that clearly document the lack of efficacy and dangers of fluoride ingestion and fluoride use (see the appendix). If you live in an area where the tap water is fluoridated and you want to drink the tap water but not the fluoride, you need to use a water filter with a reverse osmosis component; carbon filters will not remove fluoride.

• **Chloride.** Do not drink chlorinated water (unless the chlorine has been filtered out), as chlorine is toxic. A simple carbon filter will remove chlorine from tap water.

## PUTTING TOGETHER A HEALTHFUL DIET

If you look at the items in the two preceding lists, you can see that I'm not asking you to consider a radical eating plan, but a sensible, diversified one that leaves you plenty of room to include your personal favorites. Now here are some tips on how to enjoy them:

- Eat three or more times a day. This helps keep your blood glucose levels stable and thus helps avoid fatigue and mood swings. Some people find that five or six small meals—some of which may include little more than an apple or a few whole wheat crackers with natural peanut butter—works best for them. Others function best with three substantial meals and perhaps a small snack. Experiment to find the approach that makes you feel best.

- When practical, eat your fruits and vegetables raw or lightly steamed. Season the vegetables with herbs, spices, lemon, extra-virgin olive oil, or expeller-expressed olive, sesame, or flaxseed oils. Strive to include a raw vegetable salad daily made with organic ingredients.

- Prepare meats, poultry, and fish by roasting, broiling, steaming, poaching, or baking, not frying. Grilling is okay, but do not cook until charcoal forms on the food.

- Eat an optimal amount of high-quality protein, which should equal at least 15 to 20 percent of your total caloric intake. Thus, if your daily calorie intake is 2,500 calories, 375 to 500 calories should be from protein. Protein sources include beans, legumes, meats, poultry, fish, eggs, and dairy products. If possible, include at

least a small amount of protein at each meal: for example, one or more eggs at breakfast, some chicken strips
in a salad at lunch, and a piece of baked tofu or beef at
dinner. When choosing these foods, follow the guidelines presented in the "Positive Foods" list.

- Include organic, complex-carbohydrate foods (if you are
able to break down starches; some people are unable to
do this easily). The percentage of complex carbohydrates in your diet may be as low as 25 percent and as
high as 70 percent. Rarely, a diet with even less than
25 percent carbohydrates may be used for specific therapeutic purposes. This amount will depend on your individual needs. Assess how you feel when you include
more whole grains in your diet. Foods in this category
include whole grains and foods made from them (breads,
pastas, and cereals), beans and legumes (good protein
sources), vegetables, and fruits. These foods are also
good sources of fiber. Strive for 25 to 30 g of fiber daily;
this is especially important for detoxification, because
toxins are largely eliminated through stool. Complex
carbohydrates are also critical because they supply
essential sugars that bind to proteins to form glycoproteins, which in turn allow cells to better communicate with one another, especially brain cells. If this
communication is compromised, so is mental and emotional health. See "Essential Sugars," page 196.

- Fat intake also needs to be individualized. For many
years, fat was considered bad, and people were constantly encouraged to lower their fat intake as much as
possible. Recently, carbohydrates (especially refined carbohydrates) have become the villain, and some experts

consider fat to be not so bad, especially if healthy fats are chosen. Again, I believe that the percentage of fat calories needs to be considered individually; the optimal amount may vary drastically from one individual to another. For some, fat intake could be as low as 15 to 20 percent of total daily caloric intake, while for others it may be as high as 60 or 70 percent. The fats should come from natural sources (not synthetic, such as hydrogenated oils and margarines), including butter, extra-virgin olive oil, and cold-pressed sesame and flaxseed oils. You should avoid processed foods, but if you do include some in your diet, read the ingredient labels for fat content and especially avoid hydrogenated fats or oils and trans-fatty acids, which are the most health-damaging fats.

- Several times a week, include some fermented foods in your diet, such as organic, fermented sauerkraut or miso. Fermentation neutralizes unhealthy substances found in beans and grains, especially phytic acid, which blocks the absorption of calcium, iron, phosphorus, and zinc; and it adds beneficial microorganisms to food, which neutralize enzyme inhibitors and break down gluten, sugars, and other substances in grains and beans that are difficult to digest. Fermented foods also increase the population of healthful bacteria (lactobacilli) in the intestinal tract, which aids digestion, relieves constipation, and is associated with a reduced incidence of infections and allergies. Examples of fermented foods include yogurts that contain active cultures, kefir, and cultured butter; miso and tempeh are fermented soy foods; sauerkraut and pickles are common fermented vegetable foods, although many other vegetables can be fermented as well. Sources of fermented foods are in the appendix.

- Use filtered water or springwater when you cook and for drinking.
- Cook using glass, stainless steel, or good-quality enamel, not aluminum or nonstick-coated cookware.

## SPECIAL DIETS

For some people, a healthy diet that helps them prevent and eliminate depression and the symptoms associated with it may look different from what we've discussed thus far in this chapter. As I mentioned in chapter 1, some individuals react to certain types of foods, and these reactions include depression, mood swings, irritability, fatigue, and gastrointestinal problems, among others.

### Looking for Food Reactions

The presence of food reactions is something we often check for at the Schachter Center, depending on the individual's history and other information we gather during the intake evaluation. Although some physicians order skin tests for food allergies, there is little evidence that routine skin tests performed by conventional allergists are of any value. On the other hand, I have found certain specialized sublingual and skin food allergy tests and treatments, as performed by some environmental physicians like Doris Rapp, MD, to be quite helpful for some patients. I have also found that some food allergy desensitization procedures like NAET (Nambudripad's Allergy Elimination Techniques, a holistic approach to elimination of allergies) that utilize principles of acupuncture to reprogram the body to not react to allergenic foods also to be beneficial for some patients. Although the acupuncturist in my practice does utilize this latter technique to help some of our patients with food allergies, I won't be discussing this technique in detail. I will, however, discuss what you can do yourself at home to deal with suspected food allergies that might be contributing to your depression. This approach involves trying certain food elimination diets that have been successful in my practice for helping some patients with depression. I highly recommend you consider them if you suspect you have food reactions.

What should you look for if you think you might be sensitive to certain foods? Here are some telltale signs and symptoms:

- Allergy symptoms, including significant weight fluctuations from water retention, changing visual acuity, dark circles under your eyes (not related to lack of sleep), mental fogginess, fatigue, irritability, various aches and pains, and hypersensitivity to noise, cold, heat, or light.
- Presence or history of atopic allergy, such as hay fever, eczema, or allergic asthma. In fact, one study found that allergic reactions to pollen also can cause significant mood changes in some people.
- Craving for or addiction to specific foods or other substances (caffeine, tobacco, alcohol).

Although gastrointestinal problems are very common among people who have food reactions, so are depression, fatigue, and panic attacks. In fact, some people who have food reactions experience little or no gastrointestinal discomfort, yet they do suffer with depressive symptoms.

It's been shown that elimination of specific food types and strict adherence to a special diet in individuals who react to certain foods can virtually erase their depression and other symptoms, as well as restore the balance of bacteria and fungi in the digestive tract and improve absorption of nutrients.

For some people, it is critical to follow these diets to the letter—even a minute amount of gluten, casein, or certain carbohydrates can be troublesome for very sensitive individuals. Others will benefit by simply reducing certain foods. I have many patients who have been overjoyed with the benefits of adopting one of these diets. You may notice an improvement in symptoms within days, or it may take weeks. If there is no improvement after about a month, you may need to try another of the diets.

## The Gluten-Free Diet

A piece of wheat toast can contribute to Rikki's depression. So can a bowl of oatmeal. That's because this thirty-eight-year-old real estate agent has an intolerance for wheat and other foods that contain gluten, a protein that has been linked to depressed mood and is found in many grain foods, such as oats, barley, rye, and spelt. More precisely, these grains contain gliadin, a component of gluten and the real culprit in gluten intolerance. Other grains such as corn and rice also contain gluten, but because they don't contain gliadin, people with gluten intolerance typically can eat them without a problem.

Some gluten-sensitive patients who are unable to completely break down the gluten protein in their guts form smaller compounds called gliadomorphins when they eat gluten. These peptide molecules are able to enter the blood circulation and eventually the brain, where they can cause a high and then withdrawal depression just like the drug morphine. A similar event occurs in some individuals who are sensitive to the milk protein casein, as they form casomorphins, which may enter the brain and also have such an effect.

Treatment of gluten intolerance is both simple and daunting: eliminating products that contain gluten and replacing them with gluten-free foods. Fortunately, gluten-free foods are becoming easier to find as food manufacturers realize that more and more people want and need them. At the same time, shopping for gluten-free foods may seem overwhelming, because you need to scrutinize food labels not only to identify blatant sources of gluten, but also to note any additives, emulsifiers, stabilizers, and preservatives that may be made with gluten. Thus, it's not enough to buy potato bread, for example; it must also be free of other "hidden" ingredients that contain gluten.

Examples of ingredients that typically contain gluten include malt, grain starches, textured vegetable proteins, grain vinegars, brown rice syrup, dextrin, modified food starch, natural and artificial flavors, hydrolyzed vegetable and/or plant proteins, and soy. These ingredients are found in many common foods. When you read labels, look for the words *gluten-free*. Don't be fooled by the words *wheat-free*, because this does not necessarily mean gluten-free. Spelt and kamut are wheat-free but contain gluten. Also look for gluten in medications and supplements, many of which have additives that contain the protein. (See the appendix for sources of gluten-free products.)

## The Specific Carbohydrate Diet

One diet that has proved successful for some of my patients is the Specific Carbohydrate Diet, or SCD, first presented in 1951. This diet has been popularized in a book by Elaine Gottschall, which was first published in 1994, *Breaking the Vicious Cycle: Intestinal Health Through Diet* (see the suggested reading list). The SCD is a modification of the gluten-free diet, but is more rigid in terms of food choices. A major difference between the SCD and the gluten-free diet is that the former focuses on carbohydrates that are not tolerated, while the latter focuses on proteins that are not tolerated. However, there is considerable overlap between the two diets in terms of foods that are not allowed. For some difficult-to-treat cases, the SCD is a lifesaver, as it has been for Melanie, whose story clearly shows the relationship between the gut, mood, and many other conditions.

Melanie is a fifty-five-year-old staff member at the Schachter Center who has seen dramatic effects since she started the SCD. Since she was a young child, Melanie has suffered with intestinal problems, and has had problems with hypothyroidism, malignant lymphoma, and irritable bowel as well. During fall 2004, she suffered from severe depression and fatigue and took some tricyclic antidepressants, which she discontinued after a few months. In January 2005, she began the SCD, and at the time of this writing had been on it for four months. Although she reports that "there was a bit of a learning curve," she does not find the diet difficult to follow. So far she has reaped some significant benefits from the diet, including improvement in mood and energy level; elimination of severe sinusitis, which she had had for eighteen months; disappearance of stomach cramps and a distended belly (although constipation is still an occasional problem); and no mucus in stools (mucus was constant and significant in the past).

The SCD is based on the fact that some people lack the pancreatic and intestinal enzymes that allow the body to completely break down (digest) starches (chains of sugar molecules) into single sugars (monosaccharides), which can then be absorbed into the bloodstream. These partially digested starches are not easily absorbed into the bloodstream and instead travel down the gut and serve as food for disease-causing bacteria and other microorganisms. These organisms, which reproduce and overgrow in the gut, release toxins and promote inflammation, causing or aggravating conditions such as ulcerative colitis, Crohn's disease, and irritable bowel syndrome. Furthermore, toxins given off by these organisms or those produced by inflammation may result in autoimmune conditions (in which antibodies attack your own tissues) and can lead to depression, mood changes, fatigue, and many other psychiatric symptoms.

The SCD addresses the lack of specific enzymes by eliminating starches and any sugars other than monosaccharides. Therefore fructose, a single sugar found in fruit, is allowed, but a disaccharide (two sugars bound together) such as table sugar (sucrose, consisting of glucose and fructose) or milk sugar (lactose, consisting of glucose and galactose) is not.

The foods allowed in the SCD are chosen based on their molecular structure and are those included in the diet humans evolved to eat millions of years ago: meat, fish, eggs, vegetables, nuts, and low-sugar fruits. On the banned list are grains and foods made from them (such as bread, pasta, cereals), starches (potatoes, corn), and legumes (with some exceptions). The allowed carbohydrates in the diet are monosaccharides (glucose, fructose, galactose), which, because they have a single-molecule structure, are sugars that don't require digestive enzymes to be absorbed by the intestinal wall. These sugars are found in fruits, some vegetables, honey, and yogurt (which must be homemade, not commercial).

Complex carbohydrates—including disaccharides like lactose, sucrose, maltose, and isomaltose, as well as polysaccharides—in foods such as bread, pasta, cereals, corn, and potatoes are mostly not allowed: They are not easily digested (because of deficient enzymes) and become food for the damaging bacteria in the intestinal tract. Corn syrup, which is found in thousands of processed foods, is also not allowed. Some legumes—specifically dried beans, split peas, and lentils—are allowed in small amounts, but only if they have been soaked for ten to twelve hours before they are cooked and the soaking water is discarded (it contains indigestible sugars).

The yogurt required by the SCD is specially made in that it is allowed to ferment for twenty-four hours to permit the bacteria in the culture to break down the lactose (disaccharides) into galactose and glucose (monosaccharides). (The process is described in the SCD book.) Some people also take a probiotic supplement (which contains friendly bacteria) as part of the diet. Overall, the SCD deprives the harmful bacteria of their food supply, which in turn helps restore bacterial balance to the gut and creates a less toxic environment for the brain and nervous system.

## The Casein-Free Diet

Casein is a protein found in milk and products that contain milk. This protein breaks down in the stomach to produce incompletely digested substances called peptides, and then into amino acids. Some people, however, are not able to completely break down casein, and the result is that some of the peptides enter the bloodstream and then the brain, where they interact with opioid receptors and affect mood and behavior. These peptides are called *casomorphins*. High levels of casomorphins have been found in people who have schizophrenia, autism, and celiac disease, and are believed to be elevated in people who have depression, chronic fatigue, and fibromyalgia.

My experience, and that of many of my colleagues, is that a casein-free diet is highly effective in eliminating depression and related symptoms in some patients. To determine if casein is contributing to your depression, try a casein-free diet. Foods to avoid include milk and all milk products (butter, cheeses, yogurt, ice cream), as well as any item that contains any of the following ingredients: milk solids, whey, sodium caseinate, lactose, sodium lactylate, lactalbumin and other names that begin with *lact*, galactose, and protein (which often refers to milk protein). You also need to be wary of the following items, which may contain dairy: margarine, soy cheese, breads, breaded foods, hydrolyzed vegetable protein (the processing phase may contain casein), canned tuna, supplements and medicines, and chicken broth.

One more caveat: "dairy-free" does not necessarily mean there's no dairy in the item. In the United States, manufacturers are not required to list ingredients that make up less than 0.5 percent (by mass) of a product. This may not sound like much, but it may be higher than you can tolerate, depending on how much of a food you eat or the severity of your intolerance.

The casein-free diet is often combined with the gluten-free

diet, as many patients who are sensitive to casein are also sensitive to gluten.

## The Elimination or Avoidance Diet

If the previous three diets do not improve your symptoms, you can try an elimination or avoidance diet. As you'll see from the explanation below, there is some overlap between this approach and that of the other three diets already discussed. Similar, also, to the other diets is the need to eliminate the named foods as completely as possible—for instance, when you eliminate eggs, you must not eat baked goods or other foods that contain eggs or egg products. Fortunately, there are substitutions you can make while you're on the diet so you won't feel deprived. Here's how an elimination diet is structured:

- Eliminate all of the following foods from your diet for at least seven days, preferably ten: eggs and foods that contain eggs; foods that contain gluten (wheat, oats, barley, rye); corn and products that contain corn; citrus; all dairy products. Substitutes for gluten and corn foods include rice, millet, potatoes, and buckwheat. In place of dairy foods, try soy- or rice-based beverages, cheese, yogurt, and desserts. Many mainstream supermarkets now carry these products either alongside the conventional items or in a natural food section.
- During the seven to ten days, keep a record of how you feel, including any noticeable change in depression, sleep problems, irritability, fatigue, or other symptoms you had been experiencing before starting the elimination program. If you feel no changes, then food sensi-

tivities probably are not a factor in your depressed mood. If there are differences, however, it's time to identify the culprits.

- At the end of the seven to ten days, return one food group to your diet every three days. Keep a record of your responses.
- After you have returned foods from each of the eliminated food groups to your diet, you should have a good idea of what the culprits are.
- During the elimination diet, keep good notes and make those notes several times a day. Carry a small notepad with you to make it convenient.

People who go on an elimination diet risk developing nutritional deficiencies, especially of micronutrients such as thiamine, niacin, iron, selenium, chromium, folic acid, magnesium, and riboflavin. It is often necessary to take supplements of these and other nutrients to maintain optimal nutrition, especially when treating depression. If you go on an elimination diet, you may benefit from working closely with a knowledgeable nutritionist.

## ESSENTIAL SUGARS

It's true: Some sugars are essential for good mood. The target of the bad rap associated with sugar is refined white sugar, the kind people routinely put in their coffee or that is found in tens of thousands of processed foods. However, there are other sugars—natural, essential sugars—that are necessary for optimal human health, and especially emotional and mental well-being. Most of them are not sweet, and you won't find them in your sugar bowl, but they are sugars you want to include in your diet.

## The Eight Essential Sugars

Our ancient ancestors evolved on a diet that was composed primarily of fruits, vegetables, nuts, seeds, and legumes—plant-based fare that was a rich source of natural sugar compounds known as monosaccharides or single sugars. Eight of the more than two hundred monosaccharides identified so far (glucose, galactose, mannose, fucose, xylose, N-acetylneuraminic acid, N-acetylgalactosamine, and N-acetylglucosamine) are essential sugars, which are necessary for the formation of chains of sugars that connect to proteins on the surface of cell membranes. These structures, called glycoproteins, are involved in cell communication, including cells in the brain and those of the immune system. These eight monosaccharides were abundant in our ancestors' diet, but only two of them—galactose and glucose—are plentiful in our diet today, thanks largely to our love affair with processed foods that contain refined sugar. Essential sugars are also lost during harvesting (especially when produce is picked before it is ripe), cooking, and preserving.

The body needs all eight essential sugars to form carbohydrate chains (in a variety of patterns) that combine with proteins to create substances called glycoproteins (*glycol* means "sugar") and with fats to form glycolipids, both of which help cells communicate with one another. Glycoproteins, for example, make up the receptors that neurotransmitters attach themselves to on nerve cells, which means these proteins are essential in determining mood. Galactose is a component of galactolipids, which help make up nerve cells.

Fucose is believed to be active in the synapses between nerve cells, while mannose appears to be important in nerve cell structure.

## How to Get Your Essential Sugars

The best and most direct source of the essential sugars is breast milk, which contains all eight. Indirectly, fruits, vegetables, grains, and legumes are also sources, as they provide starches that are acted on by enzymes to form glucose. Other enzymes then convert glucose to form N-acetylglucosamine, N-acetylgalactosamine, N-acetylneuraminic acid, fucose, mannose, and xylose. Mannose is found in broccoli, cabbage, and seeds, while fucose is a component of medicinal mushrooms (such as reishi, shiitake, and maitake), seaweed, and seeds. Xylose can be found in rye, barley, and yeast. Dairy foods are the main sources of galactose, which is converted from milk sugar (lactose) and is also a source of glucose. Other good sources of essential sugars are kidney beans, figs, brown rice, and black-eyed peas. The need for essential sugars is a major reason for you to eat a wide variety of foods of different colors and textures. Limiting your diet to only a few types of food will drastically reduce your chances of getting these sugars.

Our requirements for the essential sugars are greater than amounts that the body produces and/or can be supplied by the diet, especially when a person is ill or under stress. One reason for this deficit is that stress and environmental pollutants both take a toll on the body's ability to convert glucose into the six above-named essential sugars. Another is that people who are lactose-intolerant and therefore avoid dairy products, as well as individuals who choose to not eat dairy foods, risk being deficient in galactose. In addition, some people lack or are deficient in the enzymes that are needed to make the conversion from glucose to the other essential sugars. To convert galactose to fucose, for example, requires fifteen different enzymes. A deficiency or lack of just one of these can hinder the conversion process.

Essential sugar supplements are now part of my treatment plan for some patients. For more information on this topic and availability of supplements, see the appendix and/or visit the website www.glycoscience.org. I have discussed essential sugars in this chapter rather than the last one on nutritional supplements because I believe these sugars should be mentioned in relation to dietary principles. High protein diets with few or no carbohydrates may be dangerous because they lack essential sugars required for good health.

## DIGESTIVE ENZYMES

In chapter 2, I introduced digestive enzymes and explained their role in the digestive process and how an enzyme deficiency can occur. Your goal is to prevent or eliminate a digestive enzyme deficiency, which you can do by eating more raw foods (fresh organic fruits and vegetables, sprouted grains) and avoiding processed foods. Another option is to take digestive enzyme supplements. Oral supplements of digestive enzymes taken just before or with meals can aid digestion. Enzymes that reach the small intestine help with digestion there as well. Digestive enzymes can improve digestion of protein, which reduces the amount of undigested protein molecules that may leak out of the intestinal wall into the bloodstream (see chapter 2).

Look for digestive enzyme supplement brands that contain

enzymes that work on all three of the macronutrients (fat, carbohydrates, protein), which means the label should list at least
one each of protease, lipase, and amylase, plus enzymes to
break down milk sugar (lactase) and fiber (cellulase). Comprehensive enzymes are now available that contain disacchari-
dases, which break down disaccharides (two sugars) and are
especially useful in patients who respond to the SCD (see the
section earlier in this chapter). Some digestive enzyme supplements also contain papain (papaya fruit extract) and bromelain
(from pineapple), which work on proteins.

Some people, especially older individuals and people with
heartburn, need to take betaine chloride along with digestive
enzymes. Betaine chloride adds more stomach acid to the
digestive process. Do not take this supplement without first
consulting your physician; it is not safe if you have had any
condition associated with excess acidity.

Digestive aids, such as digestive enzymes, should also be
considered as nutritional supplements and could have been included in the last chapter on supplements. However, since they
are so intimately involved with one's diet and the functioning
of the gastrointestinal system, they are included in this chapter
on eating habits and diet.


## DRINK TO YOUR HEALTH

Water intake is critical, especially if you are going through
a detoxification program. For optimal health, the choice is
clear: filtered water and plenty of it, at least 1 to 3 quarts
daily depending on your size. If this is more than you usually drink per day, build up your water intake gradually over
a few weeks until you reach your goal. An easy way to make

sure you get enough water is to carry a water bottle with you so you can sip from it all day long. Another way to enjoy filtered water is to make herbal tea, hot or cold, and sip that as well.

Filtered water has become big business, but it's also a necessity. You can buy bottled springwater, but this is an expensive option, it's inconvenient, and it contributes to the growing problem of disposable plastic bottles. Alternatively, you could install a filter on your home water system and have healthy water available all the time. You can avoid fluoride, chlorine, arsenic, and other contaminants depending on the type of filter you purchase. There are two main types of filters. A carbon filter removes impurities but not fluoride. A reverse osmosis filter system removes most impurities, including fluoride, chlorine, and arsenic. See the appendix for a list of filter manufacturers.

## THE BOTTOM LINE

A diet that supports and promotes a healthy mental and emotional state does not have to be complicated or mundane. It should be natural and organic so you can avoid or at least significantly reduce your exposure to health-damaging toxins, and varied so you won't get bored and will supply yourself with the variety of nutrients necessary for health. The diets discussed in this chapter meets these requirements *if* you follow the guidelines. If you do, every meal you eat will contribute to good mood and overall well-being.

*Chapter 8*

---------- ❦ ----------

# Rid Your Body of Mood-Altering Toxins

Americans are obsessed with cleanliness. Antibacterial soaps, detergents, and other cleaning products are all the rage. To fuel this desire, there are more than a hundred companies in the United States that manufacture such cleaning materials, and the result is a healthy $16-billion-per-year industry that markets everything from germ-killing hand soaps to antibacterial mattresses.

Yet for all our concerns about outer cleanliness, we are falling short on inner cleanliness. Our bodies are repositories for pollutants and other poisons that surround us—toxins that can have a deleterious effect on emotional and mental functioning. In this chapter, you'll learn how to safely and effectively rid your body of the poisons that are increasingly being introduced to it through the air, water, food, and everyday items in your home, workplace, and environment. These toxins are insidious and tend to accumulate slowly in tissues and organs. Removing them, and preventing them from taking up residence in the first place, can restore physical and emotional harmony and balance to your life.

I'll discuss various toxins, as well as some seemingly innocuous substances, that can have a negative impact on emotional and physical health and explain how you can safely avoid and eliminate them from your life using techniques such as chelation, sauna therapies, and colon hydrotherapy.


## OUR TOXIC WORLD

We live in a world more polluted than that of our grandparents. Potentially poisonous chemicals infiltrate every corner of our lives, from the additives in our food to the toxins in common products in homes, offices, schools, and churches. No one is immune from this silent invasion. Even unborn children can fall victim to secondhand smoke, vehicle exhaust, pesticides, and allergens, as shown in numerous studies of pregnant women and their infants. These studies show, among other things, that these toxins can alter the chromosomes in utero and increase cancer risk, as well as other physical and neurological problems.

Environmental illnesses (ailments and symptoms that are associated with exposure to pollutants in the environment) are serious problems and important factors in depressed mood. Take, for example, indoor air pollution. The Environmental Protection Agency (EPA) has determined that indoor air pollution is one of the most common environmental health risks: Indoor pollution levels can be two to five times, sometimes even more than one hundred times, greater than outdoor levels. The sources of this pollution are items as varied as fax and copier paper, makeup, household cleaning supplies, pesticides, medications, building materials, paint, furniture, clothing, and children's toys—all sources of potentially dangerous chemicals that can be emitted into your indoor environment.

Doris Rapp, MD, an expert in environmental illness, has noted that "environmental illness can be every bit as real as that caused by germs . . . and can trigger serious physical, neurological, and psychological problems," including depression, moodiness, aggression, fatigue, and irritability. While chemicals are touted as providing us with a better standard of living, many of them are silently and insidiously breaking it down and frequently causing or contributing to depression—literally right under our noses.

You can fight back by avoiding harmful substances whenever possible and finding effective ways to eliminate them from your environment and body. Let's look at some of the strategies here.

## NATURAL DETOX: YOUR BODY AT WORK

The human body has its own protective barrier system as well as its own cleaning or detoxification system, which is always at work more or less efficiently, depending on numerous factors that I discuss below. Let's see how it works and what you can do to facilitate the process.

### The Body at Work

The human body is constantly engaged in activities that prevent toxic substances from entering it and allow it to purge itself of waste materials. The main protective barriers are the skin and mucous membranes of the gastrointestinal and respiratory systems. Despite these barriers, toxic substances get into the body. The body attempts to prevent these toxins from interfering with vital processes by sequestering them in structures related to the immune system, such as the lymph nodes and the spleen, or in connective tissue structures, like bone, ligaments, tendons, muscles, and fat. When these structures become saturated, symptoms of toxicity occur.

The main forms in which waste is eliminated are stool, urine, sweat, saliva, and carbon dioxide (from the lungs), and each is capable, to varying degrees, of transporting toxins from the body. For natural detoxification to occur, it's necessary for each of the systems responsible for delivering waste products to operate optimally.

Optimal urine and sweat production and elimination, for example, depend on adequate water intake (see chapter 7); sufficient intake of fiber, water, and oils is necessary for efficient and daily elimination of stool. Although the American Gastroenterological Association states that the normal number of bowel movements differs from person to person, from as many as three per day to only three per week, I believe that at least one per day is preferable, with two or three being the goal. One way to complement cleansing of the bowel is through colon hydrotherapy, which I talk about later in this chapter. Release of toxins through sweat can be enhanced through exercise and use of saunas, which are also discussed in this chapter. Exercise and deep breathing techniques help the body to eliminate carbon dioxide and are also effective ways to treat depression. They are discussed in chapter 10.

Toxins in the body need to be processed before they can be removed. The organ primarily responsible for preparing waste products for their final exit is the liver.

**The Liver at Work**

The liver is a real workhorse: Every minute it processes about 2 quarts of blood, which in an adult is equal to about 25 percent of the body's total blood supply. This hardworking organ performs several critical functions, but here we will concern ourselves with how it processes health-damaging substances so they can be safely and efficiently eliminated from the body. This function can be broken down into two main phases:

• **Phase 1.** During this phase, fat-soluble toxins (most are fat-soluble) that have been transported to the liver via blood and lymph are oxidized with the help of a group of enzymes called P-450, so they can be converted to water-soluble substances in phase 2. This process readies the toxins for more efficient removal from the body.

• **Phase 2.** The newly oxidized toxins are bound with any of several substances, including glutathione, glycine sulfate, and glucuronate, to make them water-soluble and easier to eliminate either through the kidneys or through the bile, which is eliminated with the stool. Toxins that are not fat-soluble or that are partially water-soluble in their original state when they reach the liver skip phase 1 and pass directly to phase 2.

Effective detoxification depends on both phases operating at their best, and various factors wield an influence on this process, including age, hormone levels, heredity, lifestyle, gastrointestinal health, and nutritional status. Although you can't change your age, you can have an impact on the others. In fact, the hormonal, nutritional, lifestyle, and gastrointestinal health recommendations discussed elsewhere in this book promote liver health. In particular, it's important to mention some of the nutrients the liver needs to conduct phase 1 and 2 detoxification. Without proper nutritional support, the liver is unable to help the body rid itself of dangerous toxins. (Also see chapter 7.)

First on the list of critical substances is glutathione, an antioxidant that binds itself to toxins and helps transport them from the body. Glutathione is a natural *chelator* that is involved in a process known as *chelation*, which I discuss on page 221 (see "Chelation"), along with more about glutathione. Other antioxidants that facilitate liver detoxification include vitamins C and E, selenium, N-acetylcysteine (NAC), and beta-carotene. Cofactors that are also needed include riboflavin, niacin, magnesium, iron, and various phytonutrients, such as indoles (found in cruciferous vegetables like cabbage, brussels sprouts, broccoli, and cauliflower) and quercetin (found in apples, red grapes, red wine, onions, and other foods). The amino acids methionine, glycine, cysteine, glutamine, taurine, and aspartic acid are especially helpful, so it's important to consume a sufficient amount of protein each day (see chapter 7). Another nutrient, calcium d-glucarate, is found naturally in certain fruits and vegetables and can also be taken as a supplement. Optimal detoxification also depends on proper hydration, so make sure to drink six to eight glasses of pure water daily.

## HEAVY METALS AND OTHER ENVIRONMENTAL TOXINS

Heavy metals, such as mercury, lead, cadmium, and arsenic, as well as chemical toxins, pesticides, and other environmental poisons, can have a dramatic impact on physical, emotional, and mental health. Once these poisons invade the body, they settle into tissues and promote the formation of *free radicals*, unstable molecules that damage cells and organs. The result can be depression, fatigue, joint and muscle pain, dizziness, memory problems, headache, hyperactivity, and neurological disorders, among other symptoms.

You may say, "I don't work in a factory or chemical plant, so I'm not exposed to these toxins," or "I'm very careful about using chemicals in my home," and believe you and your family are not affected by environmental poisons to any appreciable degree. Yet the ubiquitous nature of these damaging substances makes it necessary for you to always be conscious of where they are in the environment, how to avoid them, and how to eliminate those that have harbored themselves in your body. It's also true that the impact of toxins differs from person to person, depending on an individual's general state of health, heredity, lifestyle, dietary habits, and age. But everyone is affected at some level by these toxins, and their impact can grow more pronounced over time if exposure to the substances continues and/or deposits in the body are not eliminated. The body works very hard to deal with and eliminate these poisons, but the task can be overwhelming for some individuals, who can then suffer with any number of symptoms.

I am reminded of Olivia, a forty-three-year-old marketing analyst who has chemical sensitivities to various substances, including formaldehyde. Exposure to this chemical, especially when she goes into an area in which it may be concentrated—such as clothing or fabric stores (permanent press fabrics are treated with formaldehyde), or stores that have furniture (formaldehyde is used in processed woods)—causes her to become very depressed and experience auditory hallucinations.

Her pronounced chemical sensitivity even made it difficult for her to work in an office building, so she works at home and goes to the office only a few hours a week for meetings.

We significantly improved Olivia's condition by having her participate in a detoxification program, which includes taking nutrients, such as niacin and vitamin C, that help the body rid itself of organic toxins like formaldehyde. She also takes low-heat saunas to help eliminate the toxins through perspiration. After a few weeks of daily saunas and nutritional therapy, she can much better tolerate environments in which formaldehyde is present, although she is still sensitive to the chemical.

Naturally, not everyone who is exposed to formaldehyde experiences these symptoms. But people can and do react to environmental toxins and do not realize that their depression and related symptoms are a result of their exposure. Fortunately, there are ways we can test for such sensitivities.

## Testing for Environmental Toxins

The heavy metals most often detected in the body at potentially damaging levels are aluminum, arsenic, cadmium, lead, mercury, nickel, and tin. Three of these—arsenic, lead, and mercury—are most often associated with depression and mood disorders. One test used to detect levels of heavy metals involves collecting urine for six hours after ingesting dimercaptosuccinic acid (DMSA), an oral chelating agent (see "Chelation" in this chapter). The patient then sends a sample of the urine to a laboratory to test for toxic minerals. The red blood cell mineral test can also be used to measure toxic minerals.

**Mercury and the Amalgam Dilemma**

It's a well-known fact that Abraham Lincoln took a little "blue pill" as a treatment for melancholy. That little pill contained elemental mercury, a neurotoxin that can cause serious neurological symptoms, including depression, dizziness, sudden outbursts of rage, chronic headache, and memory deterioration. Fortunately, Mr. Lincoln recognized the effects of the pills and stopped taking them before his inauguration.

The lack of little blue pills on the market today has not eliminated exposure to mercury, which continues to be a common and serious problem in the United States. In fact, millions of people are exposed to mercury every day in the amalgam ("silver") fillings in their mouths. Although this is slowly changing (as a result of lawsuits and new information), the American Dental Association (ADA) has maintained over the years that amalgams, which contain at least 50 percent mercury, are safe for patients. Yet at the same time, the ADA's Council on Dental Materials warns dentists that vapors emitted from scrap amalgam are extremely dangerous, recommending that dentists and dental personnel use a no-touch policy when handling amalgam and that mercury be stored in tightly sealed containers. The question, of course, is how mercury can be considered dangerous for dental office workers yet safe to put in your mouth, as the ADA insists.

The ADA argues that once the mercury-containing amalgam fillings are placed in the mouth, no mercury is emitted from them. This statement is patently false, as we have demonstrated with many of our patients who have been tested by biologically oriented dentists. Basically, a device measures the ambient mercury concentration in the air in the mouth. Then the patient chews gum for ten minutes. Immediately afterward, the ambient mercury level is measured again. Frequently, the concentration increases to levels much greater than what the Environmental Protection Agency considers safe, proving that mercury is being emitted from the fillings. Other studies clearly show a relationship between the number of amalgam fillings in the mouth and the amount of mercury excreted in urine, and that these fillings cause or contribute to symptoms such as depression, irritability, loss of memory, muscle weakness, chronic diarrhea and/or constipation, chronic headache, allergies, and muscle pain. Long-term, chronic low-dose mercury, for example, such as that which leaks from amalgams, causes mood, memory, and neurological problems, according to dozens of studies.

Amalgam fillings can emit mercury vapors when you chew, grind your teeth, or drink hot liquids. Research shows that one amalgam may release from 1 to 19 mcg of mercury daily into the body through these actions. The vapors are absorbed through the mucous membranes in the mouth and can cross the blood–brain barrier, affecting the brain and other nerve tissues. This action continues *throughout the entire life of the fillings.* Many studies show that even very low levels of mercury exposure, commonly experienced by people with amalgam fillings, are sufficient to cause depression, and that these people have significantly more neurological, memory, and mood problems than people without amalgams. Of interest is that depression and suicide rates in dentists are much greater than in the normal population and may be a reflection of their lifetime exposure to mercury.

In 1994, the US Public Health Service established a safe level of amalgam mercury chronic and acute exposure at

0.28 mcg per day. This means that even at the low end of the range (1 to 19 mcg per day per filling), individuals who have only one amalgam are exposed to at least nearly four times the level of mercury deemed "safe" by the US government. Since the average adult has eight amalgams, the potential exposure rate is dramatically higher.

## What to Do with Amalgams?

The issues surrounding mercury and amalgams include how to avoid amalgams, whether you should have them removed, and how mercury that leaks from amalgams can be eliminated from the body. Let's take the easiest issue first—avoidance. A relatively nontoxic alternative to amalgams is a composite, which is widely available although a bit more costly and somewhat less durable than mercury-amalgam fillings. If you or a loved one needs a dental filling, ask for a composite.

But say you already have one or more amalgams and you're worried about having mercury in your mouth. Should you have the amalgams removed? This is a question some patients ask, and it requires careful consideration. While allowing the mercury to remain in your mouth poses a hazard, so does removing it. As long as amalgams are in the mouth, they can leak mercury. Many people who have had their fillings removed report a reduction of symptoms of depression, fatigue, chronic pain, and other symptoms. The benefit is to stop the long-term exposure and absorption of mercury into your body.

The downsides of removing amalgam fillings are the cost, the possibility of absorbing excessive mercury into the system while removing the fillings and possibly precipitating an exacerbation of symptoms, and the time to go through the procedure.

Several tests are available to help make this decision. One test, the ambient mercury concentration test described above, can be done easily and painlessly in your dentist's office and may help you decide if you want to have the fillings removed.

If you decide to have your amalgam fillings removed, go to a biologically oriented dentist who is familiar with their safe removal. Chelating supplements and/or medications should be taken before and especially after the removal of the fillings. Examples of supplements that can be used are discussed later on in this chapter. The dentist should use a rubber dam in your mouth, and there should be continuous careful suctioning to help avoid the absorption of mercury released during the procedure. Several dental organizations list dentists who are familiar with the procedures. If you need help finding a practitioner who is familiar with amalgam removal, see the appendix.

## Mercury and Fish

Mixed messages about the benefits and dangers of eating fish have led many people to wonder if they should eat fish at all. On the one hand, you hear reports from the Food and Drug Administration and the American Heart Association (AHA) that you should eat fish several times a week because it's an excellent source of healthy omega-3 fatty acids and protein. On the other hand, you are warned about high levels of mercury, PCBs, and other toxins in fish, with special warnings targeted toward women of childbearing age and young children. In 2004, for example, the FDA warned that children and pregnant and breast-feeding women should eat no more than 6 ounces of albacore tuna per week. However, this warning hardly seems adequate given that tuna contains significant amounts of mercury. Men have been warned as well: In April 2004, the AHA reported on a twelve-year study in which men with high levels of mercury had a 60 to 70 percent increased risk of coronary heart disease. So what should you do?

Although the AHA recommends eating two servings per week of selected fish that typically have negligible amounts of mercury, including mackerel, lake trout, sardines, herring, albacore tuna, and wild salmon, I question this recommendation. At my center, we use the RBC mineral test and/or the DMSA challenge to test nearly all of our patients for mercury. Patients who eat tuna twice a week invariably have high mercury levels. If you are eating a fair amount of fish, I suggest that you have your mercury levels checked. To learn about how much mercury may be in the fish you choose, visit the following FDA website: www.cfsan.fda.gov/~frf/sea-mehg.html. As you will see, sample variability is significant, and sampling is limited.

If you eat fish, you should take nutritional chelators between meals, especially meals that include fish, to try to remove any mercury that enters your body. You could also eliminate fish from your menu and take toxin-free fish oil supplements, though this would provide only some of the benefits of fish. If you want to avoid fish altogether but are concerned about getting a sufficient amount of omega-3 fatty acids, you can opt for flaxseed or flaxseed oil (see chapter 5).

## Mercury and Vaccines

The major source of mercury contamination in young children, especially during the past fifteen years or so (until very recently), has been the increased exposure to vaccines containing thimerosal as a preservative. Thimerosal contains mercury and has been used routinely in most vaccines—but not the MMR (mumps, measles, rubella)—for many years. We find thimerosal, for example, in the DPT, hepatitis B, chicken pox, and all flu vaccines. This has been a very controversial topic because of the enormous social, economic, and political implications of the government having recommended vaccines that many argue have contributed to the tremendous increase in autism, ADHD, and many other chronic diseases in children that have occurred since the vaccines were introduced.

Following a report by the Institute of Medicine (IOM) in 2001, physicians now administer thimerosal-free vaccines to children six years old and younger. Nevertheless, a more recent report by IOM in 2004 suggested that there was no link between autism and other problems and vaccines, and that no further research should be done. The National Vaccine Information Center strongly criticized this report and said that it seriously jeopardized IOM's credibility to conduct independent, unbiased analyses of vaccine risks. If, in fact, the vaccines containing mercury have contributed to cognitive, behavioral, and mood problems in children, it is likely that these same problems carry over into adolescence and adulthood. You can find an excellent, balanced review of this entire subject in David Kirby's best-selling book *Evidence of Harm: Mercury in Vaccines and the Autism Epidemic: A Medical Controversy.* For more information on this topic, see the appendix and suggested reading list.

As of this writing, some reports suggest that following the removal of mercury-containing thimerosal from most vaccines, the incidence of autism and other neurological conditions in children has started to decline.

## Other Mercury Sources

Other sources of possible mercury contamination include mascara (especially waterproof), contact lens solution, fabric softeners, batteries with mercury cells, floor polishes, wood preservatives, adhesives, fungicides for lawns and plants, calamine lotion, tap water, and numerous other medications other than vaccines.

Occupational exposure to mercury can be a concern if you are a dentist or work in a dental office. You also may be exposed to mercury if you work in any of these areas: the manufacture of batteries, fireworks, fluorescent or neon lights, fur, ink, paint, paper, jewelry; or if you are a photographer, farmer, embalmer, taxidermist, or electroplater.

## Other Heavy Metals and Toxins

In addition to mercury, several other heavy metals can cause or contribute to depression. If you are depressed and have not been evaluated for heavy metal toxicity, you should ask your health-care practitioner for a test (see chapter 3).

### Arsenic

This heavy metal is poisonous whether it is ingested or inhaled. A major environmental source is pollution and residue from copper-smelting factories. Other sources include insecticides, herbicides, wood preservatives (found extensively in children's playground toys), ceramics, paint, tobacco smoke, and tap water.

## Aluminum

Aluminum allows potentially harmful molecules to cross the blood–brain barrier and affect neurotransmitter activity. It is found in tap water, baking powder, household pots and pans (acidic foods such as tomato sauce, as well as fluoridated water, leach the aluminum out of cookware), maraschino cherries, dental amalgams, cigarette filters, tobacco smoke, and some antiperspirants, stomach antacids, toothpastes, and laxatives.

## Cadmium

Exposure to cadmium can come in the form of tap water, cigarette smoke, evaporated milk, paint pigments, colored plastics, silver polish, fertilizers, fungicides, rubber, and rubber carpet backing. Zinc deficiency exacerbates cadmium toxicity, and the latter worsens zinc deficiency.

## Copper

The most common source of copper poisoning is water from copper pipes or from water systems that have been treated with copper sulfate. Some people unintentionally take relatively high amounts of copper (more than 5 mg per day) in their supplements. Other sources of copper include copper cookware (which can leach the mineral into food), fungicides that contain copper sulfate, and cigarettes. If you are taking estrogen in the form of oral contraceptives or hormone replacement therapy, or if your estrogen levels are naturally high, you may have elevated copper levels as well.

On the other hand, copper is an essential mineral, and deficiency may also contribute to depression (as well as cardiac arrhythmia, insomnia, high cholesterol, aneurysms, and seizures). It is sometimes difficult to determine whether a person has excessive copper or a deficiency because copper is stored in the liver, and when an inflammatory process occurs, it's released into the bloodstream to prevent damage from the inflammation. Therefore, a person may have a high serum copper level, but the body may actually be deficient. Thus, clinical judgment and experience, a history of exposure to excessive levels of copper or zinc, the use of energy diagnostic techniques, and possibly a therapeutic trial may be helpful in evaluating for copper deficiency and toxicity.

## Lead

An estimated one million Americans are exposed to excessive levels of lead on the job, via fumes or fine dust from the manufacture or handling of ammunition, storage batteries, cables, pottery glazes, insecticides, processed metals, and other sources. Millions more come into contact with lead daily in other areas of their lives, such as exposure from paint (interior paints older than 1978, which can be found in old buildings, as well as the lead-based coating on old bathtubs), food cans with lead seams, meat and milk from animals that have been fed lead-contaminated feed, and airborne lead from coal burning.

At least one expert, geologist Claire Patterson, PhD, believes everyone has a subclinical level of lead poisoning because the amount of lead in modern people's bodies is about one thousand times the amount present in our ancestors five hundred years ago. There is also reason to believe that people born before 1960 contain an accumulation of lead in their bodies, especially in bone marrow, stored for many years and, perhaps, causing or contributing to depression and other symptoms.

## Chemicals

There are approximately sixty thousand household, industrial, and agricultural chemicals to which you can be exposed. Many of them, when inhaled, absorbed through the skin, or accidentally swallowed, can be linked with neurological effects, causing and contributing to depression, headache, dizziness, anxiety, hyperactivity, irritability, memory loss, mood swings, muscle weakness, and incoordination, among other symptoms. It's even been shown that chronic air pollution (especially sulfur dioxide) can cause feelings of hopelessness.

Some of the biggest offenders are common items: natural gas (used in most gas stoves, ovens, and water heaters) and oil, and volatile organic solvents, which are found in products such as paint, fresh newsprint, permanent-ink pens and markers, glues, cleaning products, cheap perfumes, disinfectants, pesticides, varnishes, and paint thinners. The ingredients in these products, such as carbon disulfide, cresol, toluene, and methyl chloride, can easily cross the blood–brain barrier and immediately affect the brain.

Other types of chemicals associated with depression are pesticides. Whether they are used on your food, on your lawn, or in your home, most pesticides are nerve poisons that can affect the nervous systems of both pests and humans. Especially harmful can be exposure to pesticides used to eliminate insects in homes, schools, and offices, because people spend a lot of time in these structures and thus expose themselves to lingering toxic residues, which can cause various neurological symptoms.

## Fluoride

It may seem odd that something as simple as drinking water can contribute to or cause depression, but it's true. And this is because of one substance that is added to the majority of municipal drinking water in the United States—fluoride.

The fluoride that is added to the vast majority of drinking water is actually hydrofluoric acid, a compound of fluorine, which is a chemical by-product of aluminum, phosphate fertilizer, cement, steel, and nuclear weapons manufacturing. Hydrofluoric acid is used to refine high-octane gasoline and to manufacture fluorescent lightbulbs, plastics, and herbicides. It is also used in toothpaste.

Fluoride inhibits the utilization of iodine (and iodide), which may be why scientific studies indicate that about 2.3 to 4.5 mg of fluoride daily suppresses thyroid activity. The average adult takes in 1.6 to 6.6 mg daily from fluoridated drinking water and other sources, according to the US Department of Health and Human Services. This amount clearly overlaps and exceeds the amount that can suppress thyroid function. This finding could help to explain why hypothyroidism, in which the thyroid is underactive or suppressed, is a growing medical problem in the United States. An estimated thirteen million Americans have hypothyroidism, whose main symptoms are depression, fatigue, muscle and joint pain, weight gain, hair loss, and other chronic problems. Many others suffer from hypothyroid symptoms although their thyroid function blood tests are normal and conventional physicians then do not diagnose the condition as hypothyroidism. For more information about fluoride, see chapter 6, and for thyroid problems, see chapter 9.

## CHELATION: GETTING THE "LEAD" OUT

Chelation is a safe, effective method designed to remove health-damaging heavy metals and minerals from the body. The word comes from the Greek *chele*, which means "claw" and refers to the ability of the molecules used in chelation therapy to attach themselves to heavy metals such as mercury, lead, and nickel and transport them out of the body in feces, urine, and sweat.

The benefits of chelation for people who suffer with depression are twofold. One, it removes harmful toxins from the body, especially from the brain and central nervous system, improves brain functioning, and results in better mental health. Two, chelation improves overall cellular nutrition and blood circulation, which results in better concentration and alertness.

Chelation is accomplished using substances called chelators, which have a special affinity for different heavy metals and minerals. Below I discuss some of the most commonly used chelators and how they work.

### DMSA

Dimercaptosuccinic acid, better known as DMSA, is a sulfur-containing molecule that has been approved by the FDA to remove lead from children who have lead poisoning. It is also used to remove other toxic metals such as mercury and arsenic from bodily tissues. Available in capsules, it chelates toxic minerals in the body and flushes them out in feces and urine.

DMSA is tolerated well by most people, but occasionally some individuals experience mild diarrhea, nausea, vomiting, appetite loss, or rash. Rarely, a condition called neutropenia (an abnormally low number of neutrophils—white blood cells that fight bacterial infections) develops. One drawback of DMSA is that along with the heavy metals, it also chelates copper, manganese, molybdenum, and zinc, and also indirectly causes low levels of magnesium, glutathione, and cysteine. Thus you will likely need to supplement with some or all of these elements when taking DMSA. Your health-care practitioner will help you with a supplementation plan.

Another chelator, an oral, injectable, and transdermal substance called DMPS (2,3-dimercapto-1-propane sulfonate), has been used by some practitioners to remove mercury and other heavy metals from the body. Unlike DMSA, however, it has not been approved by the FDA but is available from compounding pharmacies by prescription.

## EDTA

If there is a buildup of lead or cadmium in the body, injectable EDTA (ethylene diamine tetraacetic acid) may be used. Two forms exist. Calcium EDTA may be given as an injection in the muscle or by intravenous infusion. Disodium EDTA, which in addition to removing toxic minerals is capable of removing abnormal calcium deposits, must be given as a slow IV infusion. The administration of disodium EDTA either as a rapid IV push or an intramuscular injection is dangerous and should never be done. Oral EDTA is available in supplements, but is poorly absorbed, and its efficacy is controversial. For more information on EDTA chelation therapy, see the literature and articles section of our website at www.schachter center.com, as well as the website www.drcranton.com.

## Alpha Lipoic Acid

Alpha lipoic acid is an antioxidant that has two sulfur atoms; this allows it to bind with and transport metals, including mercury, cadmium, iron, and copper, from the body. Because lipoic acid can pass the blood–brain barrier, it can chelate heavy metals, especially mercury, from the brain. Once the lipoic-acid-bound mercury reaches the bloodstream, another chelator, such as DMSA or MSM (methylsulfonylmethane), can transport the toxins into the urine for elimination. The use of lipoic acid along with DMSA is especially helpful in removing mercury in children. Lipoic acid is unusual in that it is both fat-soluble and water-soluble, which allows it to work both inside and outside cells and to aid in the removal of toxins.

In many tissues of the body, lipoic acid is converted to dihydrolipoic acid (DHLA), which, like its parent, is a powerful antioxidant. DHLA enhances the effectiveness of vitamins C and E and also promotes production of glutathione (see "Glutathione," page 224).

Although the body produces its own lipoic acid, age and the presence of toxins can both cause a relative deficiency. Knowledgeable health-care practitioners can help to determine when to use alpha lipoic acid and what dosage to use. Lipoic acid is available in tablets and capsules.

One caution with alpha lipoic acid. As a result of studies done on autistic children, it appears that alpha lipoic acid, NAC (discussed on page 224), and even DMSA can nourish abnormal bacteria and abnormal yeast-like organisms in the gut. Therefore, these chelators shouldn't be used until the gut has been cleaned out and populated by friendly bacteria.

## Cysteine and N-Acetylcysteine

If the word *cysteine* looks familiar, it's because we talked about it in chapter 4 on amino acids and in the discussion of methylation and the formation of glutathione from homocysteine. Like cysteine, N-acetylcysteine (NAC) is a chelator and a precursor to glutathione. As its name suggests, it is a derivative of cysteine.

NAC is more stable than oral cysteine. NAC helps the body neutralize heavy metals, including mercury, cadmium, and lead. Supplementation with NAC is used to build up cysteine levels as well as conserve the body's supply of glutathione. To get the most benefit from NAC and to help prevent it from being oxidized during metabolism, take a vitamin C supplement during chelation therapy. A dose that equals about three times as much vitamin C as NAC is suggested. Supplements of copper and zinc should be taken along with cysteine supplements, because the latter leaches these nutrients from the body.

## Glutathione

Glutathione is a water-soluble antioxidant tripeptide that is composed of the three amino acids glycine, cysteine, and glutamic acid. This molecule has been called "the most valuable detoxifying agent in the human body." Gustavo Bounous, MD, a retired professor of surgery at McGill University in Montreal, Canada, calls glutathione "the most important antioxidant because it's within the cell," which gives it more power to influence body functioning. For glutathione to be effective, it must be in its reduced form—its two sulfur atoms must be bound to hydrogen atoms rather than to each other.

A well-functioning liver has high levels of reduced glutathione, which it needs to detoxify poisons, certain hormones, and some medications by making them water-soluble and thus easier to eliminate from the body. Low glutathione levels are associated with arthritis, depression, diabetes, heart disease, liver damage, and other chronic diseases.

Because glutathione is a natural chelator, it is typically part of a chelation program—but not directly. That's because taking a glutathione supplement, which is available in two basic forms, is often not effective. The reduced form is not well absorbed and does not easily get into cells where its action occurs, while the unreduced or oxidized form is not metabolically active. Instead, the best way to boost glutathione is for the body to detoxify, while improving methylation as discussed previously—for example, by giving methyl $B_{12}$ injections and/or taking folic acid or trimethylglycine. In addition, as previously discussed, vitamin $B_6$ encourages the formation of cysteine and ultimately glutathione from homocysteine. An improved methylation pathway assures that sufficient cysteine will be available, and since cysteine is critical for glutathione formation, this is the best way to go. Oral cysteine is usually not effective because it is generally converted to cystine, which does not form glutathione. Another way to ensure adequate levels of glutathione is to reduce toxins in the body and reduce inflammation. Adequate amounts of methionine are necessary as well, as discussed in our section on methylation. To further support glutathione production, some individuals also take whey protein, vitamin C, selenium, lipoic acid, milk thistle, and glutamine.

## Supporting Chelation Through Nutrition

It's important to maintain optimal nutrition and gastrointestinal health while participating in a detoxification program, both to facilitate the cleansing process and to help you feel your best. Chelation promotes the movement of toxins, and it's not unusual for this "stirring-up" activity to trigger some temporary discomfort, such as headache, muscle aches, fatigue, and itchiness. Depending on the degree of toxicity, these responses will disappear within a few days or weeks. You can help reduce your response to chelation and also support the process by taking the following supplements. A health-care practitioner can help you choose the most appropriate doses for your needs:

- A healthy gastrointestinal tract is essential for successful detoxification, and a test to determine its health is the comprehensive digestive stool analysis test (see chapter 3). Probiotic supplements (such as *Lactobacillus acidophilus*, bifidobacteria, and *Saccharomyces boulardii*) are often suggested to restore healthy bacterial flora.
- A nutritious (unrefined, organic food) diet is always recommended, but it is especially critical during a chelation program. This includes eating enough protein (preferably a few ounces at each meal), because sulfur-bearing amino acids (such as methionine) assist methylation and thus detoxification. Pure water is an important part of the diet as well (see chapter 7).
- Chelation can also cause the body to lose some essential minerals, so you need to take supplements to avoid deficiencies. In fact, if the body is deficient in sodium,

magnesium, zinc, and other minerals, it has more diffi-culty releasing toxic metals.

- Supplementation with antioxidants, such as vitamins A, C, and E, selenium, and zinc, benefits both the gastro-intestinal tract and detoxification.

- Many of the toxins eliminated from the body are trans-ported in stool. In fact, when chelating mercury, up to 90 percent of it leaves in feces. So it's important to maintain regular, daily bowel movements during detox-ification. Two to three bowel movements per day is the goal. If you fall short of the goal, increase your fiber in-take by eating more fresh fruits and vegetables and/or adding crushed flaxseed (1 to 2 teaspoons daily) or psyl-lium, increase omega-3 fatty acids in the form of flaxseed oil or fish oil supplements, increase your fluid intake, and consider increasing dosages of nutrients that have laxative-like effects, such as vitamin C and/or mag-nesium. Do *not* use artificial laxatives.

## SWEATING IT OUT: SAUNAS

The skin is the largest organ of the human body, as well as an effective and ready vehicle to rid the body of toxins through sweat. When the body's tissues are heated, the pores open up to healing. That's because heating the tissues enhances metab-olism and circulation and stimulates sweating. Unfortunately, many people have inactive skin, meaning they don't sweat properly or enough. Faulty sweating can be caused by sun damage, wearing tight or synthetic clothing, and repeated ex-posure of the skin to soaps, deodorants, cleaning solvents, de-tergents, lotions, and chemicals in bathing water, among other substances. It can also be caused by fatty acid deficiency, hypo-thyroidism, suboptimal iodine intake, and neurotransmitter imbalances. Repeated use of a sauna—daily or several times a week, depending on your needs and state of health—can restore the skin's ability to sweat properly and, at the same time, be helpful in efficiently eliminating damaging chemicals from the body.

Toxin-bearing cells are weaker than normal cells and don't tolerate heat well, which makes them prime targets for sauna therapy. There are several ways you can "sweat it out," which we look at here. If you have access to a sauna, are interested in using one, and don't have a medical condition that would contraindicate its use, I suggest using a sauna several times a week for no longer than thirty minutes per session, unless supervised by a health-care practitioner well versed in sauna therapy.

### High-Temperature Sauna

The use of high-temperature (150° F), chemically nontoxic saunas is the approach most people think of when they hear the word *sauna*. At this temperature, chemicals harbored in body tissues are activated and move into the bloodstream or lymphatic system, where they are transported to the liver and undergo detoxification before being eliminated from the body.

One drawback of a high-temperature sauna is that many people cannot tolerate the heat, and in fact the high temperature can be dangerous for some, including the elderly and individuals who have a heart condition, high blood pressure, or other medical problems. An alternative to a high-temperature sauna is a far-infrared light sauna.

## Far-Infrared Sauna

Far-infrared electric light sauna therapy uses incandescent infrared heat lamps or ceramic elements to deliver its healing rays. The rays penetrate the skin and heat the body from the inside, which means the air temperature can stay cooler than that of high-temperature saunas, making far-infrared saunas more comfortable and safer. There are claims that far-infrared energy penetrates the tissues deeper than traditional saunas, which allows the cells to better release damaging substances so they can be eliminated from the body. However, some scientists have questioned these claims. At present, I am investigating the relative merits of traditional saunas and far-infrared saunas and have not yet reached a conclusion about which is more effective.

## Some Sauna Guidelines

For your own safety, talk to your doctor before using a sauna, especially if you have a chronic medical condition, such as heart disease, diabetes, or asthma. Once you have clearance from your doctor, consider these guidelines:

- Your sauna session should last no longer than thirty minutes, unless supervised with careful monitoring. During your first few sessions, you may want to stay for only ten minutes and then gradually increase the time to thirty minutes over your next few sessions.
- Drink one to two glasses of pure water before you go into the sauna. Staying hydrated is very important during this process.

- After you leave the sauna, rest lying or sitting for ten minutes and drink one to two glasses of mineralized water.
- Take a cool or warm (not hot) shower and wash off the sweat with a loofah or skin brush.

Some centers make extensive use of saunas for detoxification, especially for people who have been exposed to high concentrations of toxins, such as workers in the vicinity of lower New York City after the 9/11 disaster. Such sauna sessions may last several hours and include the use of many supplements, such as magnesium, vitamin C, niacin, calcium, a mixture of oils, and other nutrients, and drinking a lot of water. Such a program was first developed by L. Ron Hubbard and is outlined in his books (see the suggested reading list).

## COLON HYDROTHERAPY

Colon hydrotherapy (colonic) is a method that introduces cleansing fluids into the colon through the rectum, followed by the release of those fluids as a way to remove toxins, impacted waste, and other health-damaging substances from the body. These substances may accumulate over time due to poor diet, improper elimination, and use of various medications.

Unlike an enema, which affects only the lower part of the colon, a colonic reaches the entire 5-foot-long colon. Colon hydrotherapy can be especially beneficial when used along with chelation or other detoxification methods, because so many of the toxins purged from the body pass out in stool.

A typical colonic takes about forty-five to sixty minutes and is painless. You may experience some mild nausea or fatigue for a few hours after the session, because toxins are stirred up in the intestinal tract. You should only use the services of an experienced colon hydrotherapist (see the appendix for a list of reference groups). Although a colonic is a safe procedure, you should not get one if you have been diagnosed with Crohn's disease, diverticulitis, hemorrhoids, rectal or intestinal tumors, or ulcerative colitis.

## THE BOTTOM LINE

Once you begin to assist your body in eliminating toxic materials, you'll discover that it's much like living in a house for a long time: You don't realize how much stuff you've accumulated until it's time to move it or get rid of it. Toxins build up in the body over time, and it takes time to eliminate them. You may also feel some ill effects from moving those toxins—temporary aches and pains—but also long-term benefits.

The methods covered in this chapter complement the body's natural detoxification process, which is spearheaded by the liver. Talk to a knowledgeable health-care practitioner about these cleansing methods before you decide to include them in your program.

*Chapter 9*

# Harness Your Hormones

$M$ost women are familiar with and appreciate the fact that fluctuations in hormone levels, especially estrogens and progesterone, can have a dramatic effect on their mood. But these are not the only hormones that can have a significant impact on your emotional and mental state, whether you're a woman or a man. That's why in this chapter we look at how sex hormones, as well as thyroid hormones, stress hormones, DHEA (dehydroepiandrosterone), and pregnenolone, impact mood and one another and how you can achieve hormonal balance as part of a treatment program for depression.

In this chapter, I'll discuss endocrine hormones produced by specific endocrine glands that secrete these hormones into the bloodstream. These hormones then may act on tissues and organs some distance from the original glands and may circulate in the bloodstream for extended periods of time. These hormones contrast with the locally active, short-lived prostaglandins discussed in the fatty acid chapter.

The human body continuously produces dozens of different hormones, and *an orchestrated balance needs to exist among these hormones in order to function optimally at a physical, mental, emotional, and spiritual level.* The best way to achieve hormonal balance is to follow the principles in this book that deal with nutrition, supplements, detoxification, exercise, and emotional and spiritual growth. Sometimes, however, it is helpful to supplement these methods with natural or bioidentical hormones, which we will discuss in this chapter. When using bioidentical hormones, it is often necessary to take more than one hormone to achieve a balance.

There are intimate relationships among these hormones. Pregnenolone, for example, which is synthesized from cholesterol, is the precursor of both DHEA and progesterone, and these are in turn precursors to other hormones, including the estrogens and testosterone. All of these hormones also have a relationship with the stress and thyroid hormones. If the levels of any of these hormones become unbalanced due to stress, illness, environmental factors, or poor nutrition, the result can be a wide variety of symptoms, including depression and other mood disorders.

Even if none of the factors I just listed were an issue, it is still a fact that as women and men age, many hormone levels decline, and lowered levels of some hormones contribute to or cause depression. Low levels of melatonin, for example, are associated with a greater risk for seasonal affective disorder (discussed in chapter 3) and moderate depression, while excessive or deficient levels of stress-related hormones (such as cortisol or adrenaline) can cause or aggravate existing depression.

If all of this sounds like a lot to digest, you're right. But I'll stick to the highlights as we explore how imbalances among these and other hormones can cause depression and mood disorders, and steps you can take to restore hormonal balance.

## STRESS HORMONES

Stress and depression often go hand in hand. Unresolved or unmanaged chronic stress can result in biochemical changes that promote and support depression and other mood disorders. Some of the changes involve hormone fluctuations, which we look at here.

### Introducing HPA

The human body has an intriguing and complex system known as the HPA axis, composed of three elements that work together to regulate the body's response to emotional and physical stress. The *H* refers to the hypothalamus, an area deep in the brain that controls hormone secretion. Any stress that lasts more than a few minutes prompts the hypothalamus to release a hormone called cortisol-releasing factor (CRF), which in turn stimulates the *P*, the pituitary gland, located at the base of the brain. The pituitary in turn secretes ACTH (adrenocorticotropic hormone), which causes an increase in the production of cortisol (a stress hormone; see the box "Cortisol" on page 235) in the *A*, which refers to the adrenals and more specifically the adrenal cortex or outer portion of the adrenal gland, which produces steroid hormones. (The adrenal medulla or inner portion of the gland produces adrenaline.) Cortisol, in turn, inhibits the release of CRF and ACTH. This feedback action by cortisol prevents excessive secretion of these three hormones and helps balance the process. The pituitary also releases a morphine-like hormone called beta-endorphin, which helps reduce pain during times of stress.

## Cortisol

Cortisol is one of several hormones in a group called corticosteroids that play a significant role in mood and are involved in how the body responds to chronic and acute stress. If you experience acute stress, the adrenal medulla produces epinephrine (adrenaline) and norepinephrine (noradrenaline), which travel to the heart, lungs, and other major muscles to prepare the body to respond to the perceived stress. The adrenal cortex secretes several different hormones, including DHEA and cortisol, which is also known as hydrocortisone.

Along with cortisol, the adrenals secrete DHEA, a critical hormone I mention here and discuss in more detail later in this chapter. The ratio of DHEA to cortisol has an impact on mood. During acute episodes of stress or illness, cortisol levels are elevated, and so the DHEA-to-cortisol ratio is low. Once the stress subsides, cortisol levels decline and the ratio increases and becomes more balanced.

Chronic stress, however, can cause cortisol levels to remain high, which can have many negative health implications, including both mild and major depression, agitation, memory problems, thinning skin, diabetes, insomnia, and osteoporosis. It also impairs the function of the thyroid hormone, thyroxine. The healthier, desired state is a DHEA-to-cortisol ratio that favors DHEA. Studies show that people can increase this ratio through stress-reduction exercises (see chapter 10), DHEA supplementation, and elimination of negative thoughts and emotions. (See "Correcting Stress Hormone Imbalance," page 237.)

Abnormally low or high cortisol levels may be found in a person with depression. If you are under severe or prolonged stress or you have undergone long-term use of cortisone therapy, your adrenals may have weakened and become unable to produce enough cortisol. Symptoms of cortisol insufficiency include depression, low blood sugar, dizziness, chronic fatigue, nervousness, headache, and gastrointestinal problems. Our goal is to achieve a healthy level of cortisol and have it in balance with DHEA.

## Chronic Stress, Depression, and HPA

With prolonged stress, the brain begins to tolerate higher and higher levels of cortisol. Over time, the adrenal glands become exhausted, and secretion of cortisol and DHEA is impaired. Animal experiments show that chronic severe stress in newborn and young rats can permanently change the HPA axis and result in increased sensitivity to stress in later life.

There is also evidence that the HPA axis is similarly affected in humans, as seen in children who have experienced childhood trauma or disruptions during early child care. In a study conducted at the University of Washington, Seattle, researchers found that children (aged seven and eight years old) of depressed mothers had elevated cortisol levels in nonstressful and mildly stressful situations when compared with children of nondepressed mothers. A review of the mothers' depression history showed that maternal depression during the child's first two years of life was the best predictor of high cortisol levels at age seven.

## Correcting Stress Hormone Imbalance

When patients show the signs and symptoms of high or low cortisol levels discussed above, I order adrenal hormone tests (see chapter 3) to get a good profile of their cortisol levels. In healthy individuals, cortisol levels are at their lowest at night (around 10 PM) and reach their peak around 7 AM.

One of the advantages of amino acid therapy is that it helps restore stress hormone balance in addition to correcting neurotransmitter imbalances. Amino acids given to increase levels of serotonin and/or norepinephrine will ultimately reverse abnormalities in the HPA axis. Other things you can do to help restore stress hormone levels include limiting your intake of sugar and refined foods, getting adequate sleep, and taking ginseng (see chapter 6).

Don't forget the power of the mind. One cause of elevated stress hormones is your own thoughts. If you entertain negative thoughts and brood about them or resort to all-or-nothing thinking characterized by anxiety and/or panic, you stimulate the release of stress hormones. Yet while the mind can get you into trouble, it can also get you out. Stress-reduction techniques, such as progressive relaxation, meditation, and cognitive-behavioral therapy, can reduce cortisol levels (see chapter 10) and depression as well.

With either high or low levels of cortisol, supplementation with low doses of cortisol can help to relieve the stress on the adrenals and promote healing. The dosage range is usually 2.5 to 5 mg given two to four times daily with an increase of up to twice this dosage under severely stressful conditions. Dr. William McK. Jefferies discussed this treatment protocol in depth in his book *Safe Uses of Cortisol*.

## SEX HORMONES

It appears to be universal: More women than men—two- to threefold more—suffer from depression. In a landmark study published in the *Journal of the American Medical Association*, researchers evaluated data on thirty-eight thousand individuals in ten countries and reported that, without exception, rates for major depression were greater for women than for men, with an overall lifetime rate of 7.4 percent for women and 2.8 percent for men. Subsequent studies have supported this higher rate among women. Although genetics and sociocultural factors likely play a role in this disparity, hormonal differences, especially the estrogens, progesterone, and testosterone, are a key factor as well. All of these hormones, which are found in both women and men, are involved in mood.

### Estrogen and Progesterone

*Estrogen* is a general term for a group of three hormones: estrone, estradiol, and estriol. Estradiol is the main estrogen produced by the ovaries and the dominant estrogen before menopause. Estrone is weaker than estradiol and is formed from estradiol. It is the most prominent estrogen in the body after menopause, when estradiol levels decline. Estriol is the weakest estrogen of the three, is made from estrone, and is produced in large amounts during pregnancy. Estrogen is also present in small amounts in men.

Progesterone is manufactured from pregnenolone, which is synthesized from cholesterol. The ovaries produce both estrogen and progesterone, and throughout a woman's lifetime, the balance between these two hormones can vary from day to day, month to month, and year to year. The fluctuations begin in puberty and stop in menopause, when the ovaries dramatically decrease estrogen production and nearly cease progesterone production. The adrenals also produce some estrogen and progesterone, and fat tissue produces estrogen in smaller amounts throughout a woman's life.

Estrogen and progesterone influence the activities of neurotransmitters and other hormones. Estrogen, for example, blocks the enzymes that break down serotonin, which allows more of the neurotransmitter to remain in the brain and act as an antidepressant. During certain times in a woman's life, however— before menstruation, postpartum, and during menopause— estrogen levels decline, sending serotonin levels lower as well, and mood along with them. Progesterone, according to Norman Shealy, MD, PhD, is a "major regulator of estrogen, testosterone, and cortisol . . . [and] is the most versatile hormone in the human body."

## Estrogen, Progesterone, and Depression

Millions of women don't need study results to convince them that fluctuating hormone levels have a significant impact on mood. But there is evidence to support it. According to the Harvard Study of Moods and Cycles, published at the 2004 American Psychiatric Association meeting, for example, one study showed that among 644 women with no history of depression, their risk of developing depressive symptoms upon entering perimenopause was three times greater than premenopausal women of the same age. Perimenopausal women who had vasomotor symptoms (such as hot flushes, hot flashes, and night sweats, which occur in about 85 percent of perimenopausal women) had more than six times the normal risk.

In 2004, researchers at the University of Pennsylvania School of Medicine in Philadelphia reported the results of their four-year study of the associations among hormones, menopause, and depression. They found that among more than four hundred nondepressed women aged thirty-five to forty-seven, there was an increased likelihood of depressive symptoms during the transition to menopause (perimenopause) and a decreased likelihood after menopause. They concluded that changes in hormone levels contribute to low mood during perimenopause.

Researchers are learning more about the impact an imbalance of sex hormones can have on mood and other factors in women by studying monkeys. Carol Shively, PhD, and her colleagues at Wake Forest University Baptist Medical Center have reported that depressed female monkeys have low activity levels, lack of interest in their surroundings, high heart rates, and disrupted hormone levels, all of which are known or suspected traits of major depression in women. The experts also found that the monkeys had suppressed ovarian function, even though they continued to have menstrual periods. Disrupted menstrual cycles can lead to low levels of estrogen, which is associated with an increased risk of coronary artery disease in both women and monkeys. If depressed women are also found to have suppressed ovarian function that has until now been undetected, Dr. Shively and her associates suggested that this finding could explain the relationship between coronary artery disease and depression.

The relevant research for women, however, is that there is evidence to support restoring estrogen levels to a normal range to improve mood. Three studies, for example, looked at how estrogen might impact depression in perimenopausal and post-menopausal women. The women in all three studies received estradiol through a transdermal patch. Remission of depression was 80 percent, 68 percent, and 67 percent among the treated women, compared with 22 percent, 20 percent, and 18 percent among women who received placebo.

Psychiatrist Stephen Stahl of the University of California–San Diego, has even suggested that women who are taking antidepressants need to have adequate levels of estrogen before they can respond to the drugs. Thus, in some women who are being treated with antidepressants and not responding, low estrogen levels may be one reason for the lack of response. This was the case for Margorie, a fifty-two-year-old Realtor who had tried several different antidepressants prescribed by her general practitioner over a two-year period without relief. It was only by serendipity that she found relief when her gynecologist prescribed natural estrogen to help Margorie with hot flashes and other menopausal symptoms. Within a few weeks, Margorie said she felt the depression "just float away. It was like a miracle."

Bouts of depression do seem to follow the ebb and flow of hormonal changes. According to Meir Steiner, MD, of McMaster University in Ontario, neurotransmitters may be more sensitive to high levels of sex hormones or those that are in flux, which may in turn induce depression in some women. The sudden rise in the levels of estrogen during puberty, for example, changes the sensitivity of the neurotransmitter system. Pregnancy and childbirth both cause significant changes in both estrogen and progesterone levels, while menopause is marked by a decline in both estrogen and progesterone. All of these hormonal changes may increase a woman's vulnerability to depression.

## Natural (Bioidentical) Versus Synthetic Hormone Replacement Therapy

For some women, treatment with natural estrogen and/or progesterone helps relieve depression. Before prescribing any type of hormone replacement, however, I usually recommend testing hormone levels. Identifying levels of estrogens, progesterone, and testosterone (discussed on page 245) using blood and/or saliva testing is pretty much standard in my practice, especially for depressed perimenopausal and postmenopausal women. I believe the safest and most effective way to restore estrogen-to-progesterone balance is to use natural hormones (also called bioidentical hormones, because these are hormones that have exactly the same biochemical formula as the ones made in the body).

A great deal of confusion exists within conventional medicine with regard to natural progesterone and synthetic progestins. The biochemical formula of synthetic hormones differs enough from the bioidentical formula to qualify for a patent. Under the influence of pharmaceutical companies, conventional medicine has generally prescribed synthetic sex hormones, implying that there is no difference in terms of safety and effectiveness between bioidentical and synthetic hormones. A recent large-scale study, which showed that women receiving synthetic hormone replacement therapy had higher incidences of breast cancer, strokes, and overall mortality, shocked the conventional medical community and resulted in a drastic reduction in synthetic hormone prescriptions. My colleagues in alternative medicine were not at all surprised by these results; we had been advocating the use of bioidentical hormones over synthetic hormones for years. Unfortunately, even today, many physicians fail to distinguish between bio-identical progesterone and synthetic progestins, but this is changing. Common sense and studies on bioidentical hormones suggest that these hormones are safer and more effective than the synthetics, although there probably will never be a full large-scale study of this issue given the cost of such a study and the lack of financial incentives, since bioidentical hormones are not patentable.

Natural progesterone is derived from wild yam and is available over the counter as a transdermal cream that is applied to the skin. It is available in health food stores, but the quality control on some of these preparations is not very good, which is why I recommend getting natural progesterone either from a compounding pharmacy (see page 244) or from certain reliable over-the-counter suppliers of the transdermal cream.

The usual dosage of the transdermal cream is 15 to 25 mg of progesterone applied to the skin, usually twenty-five days a month, although some protocols use progesterone during only half the month, attempting to mimic the menstrual cycle. You should discuss the best approach for you with a knowledgeable health-care provider—each has advantages and disadvantages.

In December 1998, the Food and Drug Administration approved an oral micronized progesterone for postmenopausal women. (*Micronized* means it is in a form that is easier for the body to absorb.) Physicians can prescribe this bioidentical progesterone, brand name Prometrium, and patients can obtain it in any pharmacy, though the available dosages are somewhat limited. Bioidentical estrogen is also available in oral form, transdermal patch, and suppository.

Of interest is that oral contraceptives (which usually contain synthetic estrogens and progestins) block ovulation, which results in women not producing enough natural progesterone during that month. Progesterone has many protective functions in the body, and the use of oral contraceptives will result in a progesterone deficiency. The lack of natural progesterone along with the use of synthetic progestins probably account for the increased risk of blood clots, strokes, and other serious side effects such as depression that are often seen in young women who take oral contraceptives. Generally, I advise my depressed female patients to stop oral contraceptives and find an alternative method of contraception. For women who take oral contraceptives to regulate their periods, I also recommend they switch to bioidentical hormones such as natural progesterone if needed.

## Compounding Pharmacies

Today, the vast majority of prescriptions are filled by pharmacists who read patients' prescriptions, add the prescribed amount of medication to a container, and make an appropriate label. Most pharmacists are not really involved in preparing medications.

Compounding pharmacies, however, specialize in preparing medications according to a physician's specific instructions. I use the services of compounding pharmacies every day in my practice. These pharmacies are very active in preparing bioidentical hormones by prescription. They will compound medications without potentially harmful additives and fill individual prescriptions that have been tailor-made for a particular patient, taking into consideration allergies or sensitivities, form of the drug, and other factors. Bioidentical hormones are available as micronized oral capsules, oral lozenges, patches, transdermal creams, gels, or oils. Many integrative, orthomolecular, functional medicine, and/or complementary and alternative physicians (these terms are basically synonomous) make extensive use of compounding pharmacies.

A compounding pharmacy can make an estrogen formulation that fits your needs, including bi-estrogen (containing estradiol and estriol) and progesterone, or tri-estrogen (estradiol, estrone, and estriol) along with progesterone. In addition, other hormones, such as testosterone, DHEA (discussed on page 254), and more, can be prepared as individual prescriptions or added to estrogen formulations.

## Testosterone

When Jerry came to my office, he looked older than his fifty-six years. His face was haggard from lack of sleep, his skin was gray, and the spare tire around his middle was "recent and unwelcome." He also complained of depression, irritability, an inability to concentrate, loss of sex drive, and fatigue. "I haven't made any significant changes in my life that would explain my feeling so bad," he said. "My job is fine, my marriage is good. I had a physical and my doctor said all I needed was an antidepressant and so he wrote me a prescription. But I don't want a drug; I want to know what's going on."

Our evaluation of Jerry revealed, among other things, a deficiency of testosterone, as well as low levels of DHEA and elevated estrogen. When I told Jerry we could help him by balancing his hormone levels, he was surprised but more than willing to start treatment, which included a testosterone patch that delivered biologically compatible testosterone to his system. In addition, we gave Jerry chrysin, a plant substance that inhibits the conversion of testosterone into estrogen and helped to bring this hormone into balance as well. Of course, we also suggested our entire program involving dietary guidelines and exercise to Jerry. Within six weeks, he was feeling 100 percent better.

Research from the Max Planck Institute of Psychiatry in Munich shows that men who suffer from severe major depression have a low concentration of testosterone. When comparing men with depression with those who were not depressed, the investigators also found that cortisol concentrations were 68 percent higher in the depressed men, and that the higher the cortisol level, the lower the testosterone level. This is important, not only because it shows that more than one hormone level needs to be examined in people who have depression, but because these hormone imbalances have also been associated with an increased risk of osteoporosis and myocardial infarction.

## The Truth About Testosterone

Several studies show that low testosterone levels in men are associated with low mood, and that supplementation improves well-being. But this is not true just for men. Cells throughout the body have testosterone receptor sites, especially in the brain. Testosterone helps control how nerves and the heart function, regulates blood sugar and cholesterol levels, and has a role in the formation of bone and muscle—functions that occur in both sexes. You should also know that testosterone is produced in the adrenal glands as well as the testes; thus an underactive adrenal gland can aggravate testosterone deficiency in both sexes.

## Testosterone and Depression

Thus, it is not surprising that low testosterone levels in women are associated with a high risk for depression, as well as painful intercourse, increased total body fat, lack of libido, and osteoporosis. (Note, however, that normal serum levels of testosterone in men are about ten times greater than the normal levels in women.) Like men, women experience a gradual and progressive decline in blood levels of testosterone; in women it begins around age twenty and continues until they reach menopause, after which testosterone levels remain relatively constant. High levels of the hormone can increase a woman's risk for depression as well. In contrast, women who have an excess of testosterone often have ovarian cysts, excessive body and facial hair, acne, and an accumulation of fat in the abdominal area. Because testosterone levels rise both before and after a woman gives birth, high levels may be responsible for postpartum depression. So a balance of testosterone—or any hormone—is necessary. The adage "If a little is good, more is better" definitely does not hold in the case of hormones. To achieve hormonal balance, testing hormone levels can be quite helpful, along with noting signs, symptoms, and clinical response to treatment.

Perimenopausal and postmenopausal women who are depressed experience enhanced mood and energy when they take testosterone along with estrogen. If you are a woman and you and your physician decide that testosterone may improve your mood, it's important to carefully determine the optimal dose, because this hormone can stimulate male-like characteristics, such as deepening of the voice and the appearance of facial or body hair. Natural testosterone can be included in an estrogen-progesterone formula prescribed by your physician and prepared by a compounding pharmacist. Natural testosterone is also available alone as a cream and an oral micronized capsule.

## THYROID HORMONES

If you're looking at the Symptom Profile for thyroid dysfunction and nodding, you have a lot of company. According to the Thyroid Society, 10 to 15 percent of people who are depressed have hypothyroidism (low thyroid hormone production) and, conversely, most people who have hypothyroidism are depressed. Indeed, hypothyroidism is one of the most underdiagnosed conditions in the United States.

Hypothyroidism is characterized by low energy and fatigue, especially in the morning, as well as depression, difficulty losing weight, headache, brittle nails, slowed thought processes, a sensation of coldness (especially in the hands and feet), chronic constipation, fluid retention, and dry, coarse skin. An underactive thyroid can also cause stiff joints, muscle cramps, shortness of breath on exertion, menstrual irregularities, chest pain, and PMS. People with hypothyroidism may have many or a few of these symptoms.

### About the Thyroid

Located in the front of the neck just below the voice box, the thyroid gland consists of two small lobes that are connected. It is responsible for the speed of metabolic processes throughout the body; if it is not functioning properly, organs become infiltrated with metabolic wastes and sluggish.

When the thyroid gland is working properly, it uses tyrosine and iodine to make the thyroid hormone thyroxine, or T4, so called because it contains four iodine atoms. Those suffering an iodine deficiency develop an enlarged thyroid gland (called a goiter) and symptoms of hypothyroidism. The other important thyroid hormone is triiodothyronine or T3, which has three iodine atoms. Triiodothyronine is the major active thyroid hormone, being much more active than T4. T4 is produced within the thyroid gland and is later converted to the active T3 outside the thyroid gland. (See chapter 6 for more about iodine.)

Under certain conditions, such as stress, the thyroid gland may produce sufficient amounts of T4 to obtain normal thyroid blood tests, but its conversion to T3 may be inhibited, causing a relative insufficiency of active T3. In this case, a patient will have hypothyroid symptoms despite normal thyroid blood tests. This fact results in many missed diagnoses of an underactive thyroid. Overproduction of thyroid hormone, hyperthyroidism, may also have depression as one of its symptoms.

Unfortunately, many people who seek treatment for depression do not undergo thyroid testing, which means that many cases of frank hypothyroidism that could be proven by blood tests are overlooked, and the patients end up receiving inappropriate, ineffective treatment. In addition, the usual thyroid blood tests are often not sensitive enough to detect a functional thyroid deficiency. Therefore, sometimes it's necessary to try medication when the symptoms and low basal temperatures suggest a functional thyroid deficiency. However, although this has been the policy of the Schachter Center for many years, new information about iodine discussed in chapter 6 has led to a recent change in policy; now we would not prescribe thyroid hormones until iodine is tried first.

Prior to the implementation of our new policy, we evaluated and treated Andrea. When she first came to see me, this thirty-one-year-old mother of one and part-time florist reported that she was always tired, had gained 20 pounds even though she was very careful about what she ate, had chronic constipation, and didn't "really seem to care about anything anymore." During her evaluation, several very telling symptoms were noted, including her intolerance of cold ("I can't stand air-conditioning and bring a sweater with me wherever I go"), dry scaly skin, hair loss, and brittle nails. All of these symptoms indicated hypothyroidism and, according to our recent thinking, iodine insufficiency.

To confirm our suspicions, we conducted blood tests to determine levels of T3, T4, and thyroid-stimulating hormone (TSH), and found that her thyroid hormone levels were in the normal range. Yet her symptoms defied these results, so I placed her on a very low dose of thyroid hormone, nutritional therapy including antioxidants, and a moderate exercise program. Within two weeks of starting treatment, her depression had virtually disappeared and her other symptoms were improving. After three months, she had lost 18 pounds and was thinking about going to work full time.

Too often, conventional physicians will test for thyroid hormone levels and, when they obtain "normal" results, rule out thyroid dysfunction as the culprit. Some of these functionally hypothyroid patients, a very significant percentage of the US population, may actually be suffering from iodine insufficiency—and many are depressed.

## Thyroid Testing

Thyroid testing identifies the levels of several hormones, including T4 and T3, which are the most active of the thyroid hormones; and thyroid-stimulating hormone, produced by the pituitary gland that controls the production and secretion of thyroxine. When T3 and T4 levels rise, the pituitary secretes less TSH, which causes production of T3 and T4 to decline, restoring balance. If T3 and T4 levels fall, secretion of TSH again increases, which boosts production of T3 and T4.

Testing for T3, T4, and TSH levels is a good start if you have symptoms of hypo- or hyperthyroidism, but because the normal range for these blood tests is wide, it's possible to have thyroid dysfunction with so-called normal test results. Measurement of thyroid antibodies can provide additional information about the risk of depression and treatment prognosis. One report, for example, found that women with high levels of antithyroid peroxidase (anti-TPO) antibodies are more likely to become depressed than those without these antibodies. A subsequent study concluded that testing for antibody levels "seems necessary," especially in the elderly and in individuals who do not respond to depression treatment

While women are more likely to have thyroid hormone imbalance (especially hypothyroidism) than men are, a subgroup of women are at particular risk. Up to 10 percent of new mothers develop postpartum thyroiditis, chronic inflammation of the thyroid gland, and concurrent depression. This condition can be diagnosed with tests that check for antibodies against the thyroid. Research has shown that up to 50 percent of women who have high levels of thyroid antibodies during their first trimester develop postpartum thyroiditis and are subsequently at risk for postpartum depression. These women may be iodine-insufficient and will probably respond to iodine supplementation. Women who are significantly iodine-insufficient and then become pregnant will become much more insufficient, because iodine is preferentially transported to the fetus. As the woman becomes more insufficient, she is likely to develop antithyroid antibodies, and after delivery is more likely to develop postpartum depression.

## Thyroid Hormones in Psychiatry

In recent years, studies of depression have shown that some people who take antidepressants respond better if they also take T3. In one particular study of patients who had hypothyroidism, those who took a combination of T3 and T4 had better results in regard to mental and emotional symptoms than those who took T4 alone. Unfortunately, most patients with hypothyroidism who are treated conventionally usually take only T4. Occasionally patients are given T3 (as the medication Cytomel), which must be taken several times a day and can cause mood and energy swings. To prevent these problems, a physician could prescribe long-acting T3, which is available from compounding pharmacies. Today, however, I would certainly try therapeutic doses of iodine before prescribing long-acting T3.

## Treating Thyroid Dysfunction

In my experience and that of many other physicians, the synthetic T4 is not as effective as the desiccated thyroid (thyroid extract), which contains both T3 and T4. To treat an underactive thyroid, I recommend beginning with a low dose of thyroid extract, with gradual increases until the optimal dosage is reached. It can take four to six weeks to feel the full benefits. Generally, I start patients on ¼ grain (15 mg) daily. Then I increase the dosage by ¼ grain each week until we reach 1 to 2 grains daily. Usually the optimal dosage is in this range, although some patients need more. However, our new policy is to try therapeutic doses of iodine (along with supportive nutrients) first and prescribe the thyroid extract only if the iodine fails to get the thyroid to function adequately on its own.

In patients with weak adrenal function, a condition sometimes seen among people with chronic depression, this problem must be treated first or simultaneous to the thyroid treatment. This is because cortisol, which is produced by the adrenal glands, is necessary to convert T4 to active T3. Indications of low adrenal function include allergies, asthma, low blood pressure, breathing difficulties, skin problems, joint or muscle pain, mood swings, phobias, and weeping. My preferred approach for patients with both low adrenal and low thyroid functioning is to first try to support the adrenals with nutritional supplements, such as vitamins C and $B_6$, pantothenic acid, and adrenal extracts, while cautiously adding iodine and other support for the thyroid gland. If this fails to get a reasonable clinical response in several weeks, I then start low doses of hydrocortisone (cortisol) and thyroid extract. Nutritional support (for instance, avoiding refined carbohydrates, sugar, and caffeine, and eating whole fruits and vegetables) is recommended for everyone and is the only treatment necessary for some individuals. Although many people need to take thyroid hormones indefinitely, we are sometimes able to reduce and stop treatment as we strengthen the body and thyroid through nutrition, detoxification, and other methods discussed in this book. I also suspect that many of our patients who are currently taking thyroid hormone will be able to taper it and eventually stop it once they become iodine-sufficient.

Another consideration when treating hypothyroidism is

the need to restore balance in other areas. For example, thyroid hormone is essential for a process called oxidative phosphorylation, which the body uses to store energy by using oxygen to oxidize food. This process requires vitamins $B_1$, $B_2$, $B_3$, and $B_5$, as well as coenzyme Q10, several minerals, and other nutrients. If an individual is deficient or has low levels of these substances, then a prescribed thyroid hormone will not work optimally and may even cause side effects. Additionally, other hormones may require adjustment.

Hyperthyroidism, a much less common condition, also may cause depression. The current standard of care for this condition is surgery, radioactive iodine (to destroy the thyroid), or relatively toxic thyroid-suppressive drugs. As I discussed in chapter 6, therapeutic doses of iodine may be a safe and effective treatment for many of these cases.

Finally, because conventional blood tests are inadequate to monitor the results of treatment, the best thing your doctor can do is ask you how you feel, note whether symptoms of an overactive thyroid gland have developed, and monitor your basal body temperature.

## DHEA

Dehydroepiandrosterone (DHEA) is called a "mother" hormone because several other hormones are derived from it. DHEA is the most abundant hormone produced by the adrenal cortex. It is especially abundant in the brain and plays an important role in determining mood. In the 1950s, in fact, DHEA was studied for use as an antidepressant. Although it was shown to be effective, further research wasn't pursued until the 1980s, when interest in DHEA as an antiaging supplement exploded, and the hormone's abilities to relieve depression was noted once again. Shortly thereafter, researchers at the University of California–San Diego analyzed old data from a study that had been done in Rancho Bernardo during the 1970s and 1980s. The original study had measured the levels of estradiol, estrone, testosterone, androstenedione, DHEA, and DHEA sulfate (DHEA-S) in 699 older women. When they reevaluated the results, they found that only a low DHEA-S level was associated with depression.

DHEA is important in determining mood by itself and because it is a precursor hormone that promotes the production of other hormones involved in brain function and emotional balance. One clue that DHEA is a vital player in nervous system activity is the fact that the brain contains nearly seven times more DHEA than any other organ. Thus, a decline in DHEA levels, which begins to occur naturally around age twenty-five, could be expected to have an impact on mood and brain activity. Such thinking has fueled hopes that giving DHEA as a supplement can alleviate depression and related symptoms.

In a study published in February 2005, researchers examined whether DHEA is an effective treatment for depression that appears in midlife. Twenty-three men and twenty-three women aged forty-five to sixty-five who had major or minor depression of moderate severity were randomly assigned to receive either DHEA therapy or placebo for six weeks. After six weeks, all the participants received no therapy for one or two weeks, and then the treatment groups were reversed—the original DHEA group received placebo and the placebo group received DHEA for six weeks. Overall, 50 percent of the participants had a significant and positive response to DHEA—

improvement in depression and sexual functioning—when compared with placebo and baseline (before the study began).

## How It Works

Although it's not clear exactly how DHEA relieves depression, there are several theories. One is the fact that DHEA is the precursor for two hormones that improve mood—testosterone and estrogen. Another is that DHEA and its metabolite, DHEA sulfate, easily cross the blood–brain barrier and thus can directly impact the activity of serotonin, GABA, and other elements in the brain that affect mood. DHEA also interferes with the actions of the stress hormone cortisol, which is elevated in people who have major depression (see the box "Cortisol" on page 235), and counteracts its effects.

One goal of DHEA treatment is to restore an individual's DHEA level to the point it was at when he or she was about twenty-five to thirty years old, which is when DHEA peaks. This was the strategy in the first double-blind, placebo-controlled study of DHEA's ability to relieve symptoms in people with major depression. Patients were given 30 mg of DHEA for the first two weeks, 60 mg for the next two weeks, and 90 mg for the final two weeks. Another group of patients received a placebo. After six weeks, nearly half of the treated patients had a 50 percent or greater decrease in depressive symptoms. In another study, 90 mg of DHEA daily for three weeks significantly reduced depressive symptoms among patients with dysthymia. The response rate overall was 60 percent, which is better than the response to antidepressants for dysthymia. Most people responded within ten days.

## Using DHEA

Before starting supplementation with DHEA, your blood should be tested for DHEA-S levels or your saliva for levels of DHEA. If your levels are low and you begin supplementation, periodic blood testing or saliva levels should be done to determine whether your DHEA levels have reached an appropriate level as determined by your health-care practitioner. DHEA should not be used if you have a hormone-related cancer.

As a precaution, take antioxidants, such as vitamin E, NAC, and green tea, while using DHEA; very high doses (2,000 to 10,000 mg) of this hormone have caused liver damage in rodents. A typical dose of DHEA is 5 to 75 mg once a day in the morning. It can be taken with or without food; some people absorb the hormone better if it's taken thirty minutes before a meal, while others assimilate it better along with a fatty food. You may need to experiment to see which way works best for you.

To help ensure you are taking the optimal dose to restore your DHEA levels to youthful levels, your health-care practitioner should conduct a DHEA-S blood test three to six weeks after you begin DHEA therapy. The blood sample should be drawn three to four hours after the last dose was taken. The youthful ranges of DHEA-S are 400 to 560 mcg/dL for men and 350 to 480 mcg/dL for women, but these ranges may vary from laboratory to laboratory.

### Precautions

Before starting DHEA therapy, men should undergo a digital rectal examination and a serum PSA test to check for evidence of prostate disease, which might be aggravated by taking DHEA. That's because DHEA can be transformed into estrogen and testosterone, which can promote both malignant and benign prostate cell growth. However, there is no evidence that the hormone causes prostate cancer or benign prostate disease.

## PREGNENOLONE

Pregnenolone is produced from cholesterol and, similar to some other hormones, its production declines with age. By age seventy-five, the body produces 60 percent less than it did at age thirty-five. When pregnenolone levels decline, so do levels of other hormones for which it is a precursor, including the estrogens, progesterone, DHEA, cortisol, and testosterone. It follows that low levels of pregnenolone are associated with depression.

Pregnenolone is often touted for its ability to improve concentration and memory, but it is useful in treating depression as well. It is produced by the gonads (ovaries and testicles), adrenal glands, and liver in men and women, and is believed to prevent overactivity of GABA and other hormones that inhibit brain function. It is abundant in the brain, where it helps facilitate the transmission of nerve signals. Research also indicates that pregnenolone improves the ability to handle stress and helps protect the myelin sheath membranes, which in turn protect the neurons and brain. It also can be produced in the brain instead of being transported there from other parts of the body. This fact supports evidence that pregnenolone plays a role in brain-related activities.

Pregnenolone should be used with caution if you have a history of seizures because of its effects on GABA receptor sites. As a precursor of DHEA and other hormones, pregnenolone may increase these hormone levels and create an imbalance, causing menstrual cycle changes and interacting with hormone therapy such as oral contraceptives, which is one reason why it is not used as often as the other hormones discussed in this chapter.

Pregnenolone is available over the counter and by prescription from compounding pharmacies, as a tablet and sublingual powder. The usual starting dosage is about 30 mg daily, but higher dosages are available. Pregnenolone supplements enhance the body's ability to manufacture its own pregnenolone and progesterone, and also helps improve the function of the thyroid and other glands.

## MELATONIN

If there's one substance in the body that holds superior power over your sleep, that substance would be the hormone melatonin. And if you've ever wondered why people who are depressed are usually plagued with sleep problems, it's usually because they are deficient in serotonin, one of the main neurotransmitters associated with depression and the precursor of melatonin.

Melatonin is produced by the pineal gland, which is located deep in the brain. Exposure of the eyes to bright daylight helps to synthesize melatonin. Melatonin is then released from the pineal gland at night while sleeping in darkness. Light immediately inhibits the secretion of melatonin, and this is one reason to sleep in the dark and to avoid exposure to light if you get up during the night, which may prevent you from going back to sleep. Also, if melatonin secretion is disrupted, sleep problems, behavioral changes, and mood disorders can occur. Numerous studies have shown decreased levels of melatonin in people with depression, as well as significantly low levels in depressed children and adolescents with psychosis compared with depressed individuals without psychosis.

A melatonin deficiency can be reversed if you maintain sufficient levels of serotonin. Since this neurotransmitter is deficient in many depressed people, boosting serotonin levels with 5-HTP and/or tryptophan, as discussed in chapter 4, ultimately results in higher melatonin levels. Melatonin is also available as a supplement, usually in 0.5 mg to 3 mg doses. If you are experiencing sleep problems with your depression and the amino acids are not increasing melatonin levels sufficiently to improve your sleep, then you may need a melatonin supplement. A typical starting dose is a 0.5 mg sublingual tablet at bedtime. It is best to take melatonin for a short time only; the goal is for the body to make its own melatonin after its precursor serotonin has been replenished. After using melatonin for one or two weeks, stop taking it to see if you still need it or if you can reduce your dose. However, at 0.5 mg to 3 mg (or even higher doses), there is no evidence that longer-term use is actually harmful.

## THE BOTTOM LINE

Several specific hormones play a key role in the development and treatment of depression and other mood disorders. The fact that these hormones have intimate relationships not only with one another but also with various neurotransmitters makes successful treatment of depression more likely if you work with a physician who understands this relationship and how to prescribe appropriate hormones, amino acids, and nutrients to restore hormonal balance.

# Chapter 10

*Up with Life*

The resiliency of the human body and mind is truly amazing, and there is no question you can harness it to help you beat depression. Along with amino acid therapy, nutritional modifications, and hormone balancing, which are important parts of my treatment program, many of my patients have found that lifestyle changes, including modifications to their exercise and sleep habits, the addition of stress-reduction techniques, or psychotherapy, just to name a few, have made a significant and positive difference in their mood. Nurturing loving family relationships and other meaningful relationships are also extremely important. In this chapter, I share some of those recommended lifestyle modifications with you and tell you how to implement them.

Admittedly, when people are depressed, they often don't have the motivation or desire to make changes to their lifestyle. Generally, people prefer to find relief and cures in pills rather than in behavior modification. Yet the success of pills very much depends on attitude and actions. The most balanced amino acid and hormonal therapy plans won't provide much benefit if you sleep for only three or four hours a night, have a highly stressful job, never take time to relax, and rarely get any exercise.

In this chapter, I'll explain the benefits of lifestyle changes that, while complementary to the therapies you have read about thus far, clearly can have a positive effect on mood, and offer suggestions on how you can incorporate them into your life.

## EXERCISE: MOVING OUT OF DEPRESSION

If there were a pill that could motivate people to exercise—without any side effects, of course—I'd prescribe it in a minute. There certainly is a big need for such a product, and the inventor would probably become wealthy overnight. Alas, no such incentive is available, and so we are left with hard, scientific proof that exercise is beneficial on many fronts, including as a treatment for depression, as our motivator. And so here goes.

### The Proof Is in the Moving

Would you believe me if I told you that you could significantly improve your mood if you walk briskly or perform another form of aerobic exercise for thirty minutes a day, three to five days a week? According to researchers at Utah Southwestern Medical Center, you can. Eighty people aged twenty to forty-five who had mild to moderate depression were randomly assigned to one of five groups: two in which participants did moderately intense aerobic exercise (treadmill, stationary bike) for thirty minutes for either three or five days a week; two that involved less intense aerobics for either three or five days; or one that required stretching exercises only for fifteen to twenty minutes three days a week. After twelve weeks, people in both of the moderately intense aerobics groups averaged a 47 percent decline in depressive symptoms, while those in the less intense groups averaged 30 percent. Those who did just stretching exercises showed a 29 percent decline.

A nearly 50 percent reduction in depressive symptoms—and without the use of drugs—is a very good outcome, but how does it compare with results if you take antidepressants? A study at Duke University Medical Center looked at that question when researchers there studied 156 adult volunteers who had major depression. For four months, the individuals participated in one of three groups: aerobic exercise only, sertraline (Zoloft) therapy only, or both exercise and sertraline. The study experts assessed the presence and severity of depression in each patient before the study, after four months of treatment, and six months after treatment ended. After four months of treatment, patients in all three groups had significant improvement, but after ten months, the relapse rate was significantly lower among the people in the exercise group as compared with those in the medication-only group. Individuals who exercised on their own during the follow-up period were less likely to be diagnosed with depression.

There's yet another reason why exercise should be a part of any program to eliminate depression. Some experts say that one reason why exercise enhances mood is that it raises levels of DHEA—which, as I discuss in chapter 9, is a hormone with mood-enhancing qualities. We can take this relationship one step farther and note that exercise and DHEA, which both have positive effects on mood, are also both beneficial for the heart. It's been shown, in fact, that women with depression are at greater risk of heart attack and that exercise reduces depressive symptoms and helps improve heart health.

## Making the First Move

If there's only one thing I can say about exercise, I'd say make each session as much fun as possible. Naturally, choose activities you like and that don't breed stress. If you hate swimming, don't include it as part of your program. If you enjoy walking or jogging but don't like to do it alone, find a friend who will go with you, join a walking club, or start your own at work or in your neighborhood. If safety or transportation is a limiting issue for you, you might feel more secure exercising at home with a treadmill or exercise bike or using exercise videos.

Diversify your exercise program. Many people find walking, jogging, and/or running to be relatively easy exercises to pursue, but swimming, biking, and others that require equipment or special environments are not as convenient, and membership in a health club can be a financial burden. If you have a VCR or DVD player, you can pop in an exercise program or one on yoga or tai chi and enjoy these activities in the privacy of your own home, at your convenience. If you have access to home exercise equipment such as a treadmill, exercise bike, or rowing machine (many people own such equipment and use it as a clotheshorse; ask relatives, friends, or co-workers if they have one they are willing to lend to you), you can add some diversity to your program in this way as well.

Your exercise sessions should be a time you release stress, not add to it. But if you're someone who feels as if you're wasting time if you dedicate thirty minutes a day to a brisk walking program, you can relieve your stress *and* your depression if you take along a handheld CD or cassette player and listen to music or an instructional tape while you work out. Take along a mini cassette recorder and tape notes—letters you need to send, your grocery list, your to-do list for the day—while you're on the move.

## LET THERE BE LIGHT

Roseanne's depression arrived predictably each fall: As the days grew shorter in her Minnesota town and daylight was a fading commodity, her mood sank lower and lower. This had been her pattern for more than a decade. By the end of the year, she said her family and friends were ready to pack her away with the Christmas ornaments. "I was not very pleasant to live with," she said. "I was irritable, tired all the time, and I gained weight, which made me even more depressed. I didn't feel like doing anything, and some days I ached all over. I was miserable." Roseanne had the classic symptoms of a type of depression called seasonal affective disorder, or SAD (see chapters 3 and 6). Her husband kept urging her to take antidepressants, but Roseanne refused, arguing, "It will go away in a few months," which was true year after year.

Then one Christmas, her son and daughter-in-law gave her a light box. "They told me I should sit in front of it for up to an hour every morning when I get up," Roseanne said. "I thought they were crazy." But she tried it anyway, spending the time reading the newspaper and drinking tea. By the end of January, she was feeling so much better, she recommended a light box to a co-worker who was suffering with similar depression.

## How Light Therapy Works

Light therapy involves exposing yourself to a measured amount of balanced-spectrum light, usually at an intensity of around 10,000 lux, emitted from a light box that contains white fluorescent light tubes covered with material that blocks ultraviolet light. (For comparison, normal indoor light is about 500 lux, while standing outside on a sunny summer day exposes you to 100,000 lux.) Your eyes register the light and then send signals to the hypothalamus in the brain, where the body's clock function is maintained. The light helps synchronize your sleep–wake patterns with your lifestyle.

To get the most benefit from a light box, you should do your sessions early in the day and sit from 1 to 2 feet away from the front of the box. Keep your eyes open but do not look directly into the light. Your first few sessions should last about fifteen minutes; then gradually increase each session until you reach thirty to forty-five minutes. Some people find they can skip a day or two in succession without significant effects, but missing three days in a row causes symptoms to return.

Some people experience improvement in depressive symptoms within two to four days; others notice a change after a week or two. If you don't note an improvement after four to six weeks of treatment, you are probably not going to respond to this approach.

Although uncommon, side effects can occur during light therapy. These may include photophobia (hypersensitivity of the eyes to light), headache, fatigue, irritability, hypomania, and insomnia (if therapy is done too late in the day).

## Is Light Therapy for You?

Light therapy is safe and noninvasive, as well as an excellent complement to other therapies for depression. Its value for people who have SAD has been well documented, and a recent review of twenty controlled studies of light therapy concluded that it is effective in the treatment of nonseasonal depression as well.

Light therapy is also especially helpful in pregnant women who suffer with depression. These women are in a double bind: Antidepressants may have a negative effect on a newborn's growth and development, while untreated depression during pregnancy has been associated with premature birth, lower birth weight, childhood behavioral problems, and an increased risk of preeclampsia. C. Neill Epperson, MD, a psychiatrist with Yale School of Medicine, found that depressed pregnant women who used daily bright light therapy for ten weeks had significant reductions in depressive symptoms when compared with women who were exposed to dim light. In a prior study, pregnant women reported a 49 percent improvement in depressive symptoms after only three to five weeks of daily bright-light therapy.

Light therapy has become a popular treatment for depression, and so light boxes are widely available through the Internet, mail order, and health and medical specialty stores. The appendix in this book offers you some sources of light boxes.

To help prevent depression and increase a sense of well-being, I recommend that everyone spend an hour or more outdoors during peak sunlight, weather permitting. I believe it is reasonable to think of bright light as a nutrient, and spending time outdoors helps to supply that nutrient. For more information on the relationship between health and light, see the suggested reading list.

## RELAXATION THERAPIES

When you are experiencing physical or emotional stress, your body releases hormones that affect every cell in your body. This "stress response," also known as the fight-or-flight response, was first explained in the 1950s by Hans Selye. In the late 1960s, Herbert Benson, MD, of the Harvard Medical School, spotlighted the opposite response, the "relaxation response," which he described as "an inborn set of physiological changes that offset those of the fight-or-flight response . . . [and these] changes are coordinated [and] occur in an integrated fashion." Certain techniques, such as meditation, yoga, deep breathing, and progressive relaxation exercises, elicit the relaxation response and have a positive effect on mood. Participation in these or other relaxation therapies, too numerous to cover here, can provide a powerful boost to any depression treatment program.

### Yoga

Step back about five thousand years and practice the art of yoga as a way to reduce stress. The goal of yoga, which means "union," is to become one with your true self, but the focus of many who practice it today is stress control, improved physical fitness, and enhanced mental clarity. There are many different types of yoga; some concentrate on physical strength and flexibility, while others emphasize spiritual growth. Regardless of which yoga discipline you choose, the practice should be used to complement treatment of depression, not replace it.

Proper breathing is a critical part of yoga, and several studies have looked at the effects of yogic breathing on depression. In one study, severely depressed patients got as much relief from daily practice of yogic breathing as they did from an antidepressant; in another, the breathing exercises produced faster improvement than no treatment at all. To appreciate a very simple type of yogic breathing, see the accompanying box.

## Yogic Breathing

There are various yogic breathing techniques, but here is one of the easiest to learn.

1. Sit comfortably in a chair with your feet flat on the floor.
2. Loosen any clothing that may be tight or restrictive around your abdomen, waist, and chest.
3. Place your hands in a relaxed position on your lap.
4. Place the tip of your tongue against the ridge behind and above your upper front teeth. You should keep your tongue in this position throughout the exercise.
5. Breathe in slowly through your nose (keep your mouth closed) to a count of five. Be conscious of allowing your abdomen to expand as you breathe in.
6. Hold your breath for a count of seven.
7. Exhale slowly through your mouth to a count of six or seven. You may make a "whooshing" sound as you exhale.
8. Repeat steps 5 through 7 for a total of five breaths.

In another study, published in February 2005, investigators noted that a specific type of yoga, Sudarshan Kriya, "can alleviate anxiety, depression, everyday stress, post-traumatic stress, and stress-related medical illnesses." Researchers also found evidence of yoga's ability to significantly reduce depression and anxiety in a study of twenty-eight young adults with mild depression. Midway through the ten hours of yoga instruction done over a five-week period, individuals who participated in the yoga classes reported significantly decreased symptoms of depression and anxiety compared with controls.

If you want to include yoga as part of your program, you will need some instruction, which you can get through books, videos, community classes, or private instruction. To help you learn more, see the suggested reading list.

## Meditation

Depression is characterized by low self-esteem and feelings of hopelessness and isolation. Meditation increases a person's self-confidence, self-worth, and sense of belonging in the world. Thus it's fortunate that meditation is shedding its coat of mystery and is being accepted by the mainstream, including those in the medical realm, as a viable way to treat depression, stress, and tension. And a big reason for that acceptance is that there's scientific research into the effectiveness of meditation showing this to be true.

A review of twenty studies that looked at the use of mindfulness meditation (a form of meditation I explain on page 271) to relieve conditions such as depression, anxiety, and pain found that this approach may help many people cope with these and similar medical problems. Why does this improvement occur? Researchers at James Cook University of North Queensland, Australia, studied the relationship between various hormones and mood changes in eleven elite runners and twelve trained meditators. We know from other studies that hormone levels change after exercise, but what effect does meditation have? The Australian study showed that mood was elevated after running and after meditation, and that both groups had similar increases in corticotropin-releasing hormone levels (see chapter 9). It was concluded that both running and meditation can improve mood and that this improvement is associated with changes in corticotropin-releasing hormone levels.

Generally, there are two basic approaches to meditation: concentrative and mindfulness. In concentrative meditation, you focus your attention on something repetitive, such as a repeated word or phrase, your breathing, or an object (a lighted candle, say, or something in nature). The idea is that your concentrated effort helps you rid your mind of extraneous thoughts and to be still.

In mindfulness, you are an observer of your own thoughts, but you do not allow yourself to participate in them. Some people liken it to watching a parade going by: You acknowledge your thoughts but you stay on the sidelines and don't allow yourself to think about them.

Meditation is an effective tool in the fight against depression and stress, and it doesn't have to cost you anything except some time to learn more about it. You can learn how to meditate from books, audiotapes, videos, meditation classes, and stress-reduction clinics. See the suggested reading list for help in learning more about meditation.

## Visualization and Guided Imagery

A patient once described visualization as "a daydream that heals," an apt description for this stress-reduction method. In visualization, you allow a pleasant scene or other image to enter your mind's eye and then focus on it completely, imagining any sounds, smells, tastes, and textures associated with it. You can use visualizations to relieve stress and enter into a calmer state. Similarly, guided imagery can be described as "a movie that heals," because it takes visualization a step farther: You imagine pleasant scenes and then you take a mental trip through them, so that the images and sensory input change as you create a story or series of images that promote harmony.

If you close your eyes and visualize someone running their fingernails down a chalkboard, does a shiver run up your spine? That image elicits such a response in many people, even though it's only an image. Why? Visual, tactile, and auditory images are produced in the cerebral cortex, the thinking and language area of the brain. Experts have used an imaging technique called positron emission tomography to look at the brain and have shown that the cerebral cortex is equally activated whether people actually experience something or just visualize it in their mind. So although it might be very relaxing to physically lie on a sandy beach in the South Pacific, you can reap at least some of the stress-reducing benefits if you vividly visualize the scene and, if you wish, conduct a guided "tour" beyond it, focusing on sensory stimuli that make you feel calm.

At the Schachter Center, Peter Reznik, PhD, CSW, incorporates a number of innovative psychotherapeutic techniques, including imagery, to help patients deal with depression. He presents his approach on his CD *Staying Healthy in a Stressful World: A Comprehensive Manual for Self Mastery and Freedom from Stress.*

You can learn visualization and guided imagery using self-help books or audiotapes, or you can join a class or take private instruction. Resources for books and tapes are provided in the appendix.

## Progressive Relaxation

"The best thing about progressive relaxation is that I can do it just about anywhere," says Lynne, a forty-seven-year-old marketing analyst. "I can do simple exercises while sitting at my desk, and more involved ones at home. They help me get rid of a lot of tension and get a new perspective on my situation."

Progressive relaxation helps you focus your attention on different areas of the body in a systematic manner and progressively release tension that has built up in the muscles. The exercises are best done while lying down, although you can get good results from doing them while seated, as Lynne does. An example of a progressive relaxation exercise is below. You may want to try this one or variations on it one or several times a day to gauge how it makes you feel.

- Lie down on your back on a firm, comfortable surface, such as an exercise mat, hard mattress, or even a recliner. Wear comfortable clothing and no shoes.
- Close your eyes and allow your arms to relax by your sides.

- Take a deep breath through your nose, hold it for five seconds, and then release it slowly through your mouth. Repeat several times.
- Begin with your hands. Make tight fists and feel the tension in your hands and arms. Hold the contractions for five to ten seconds. Take a deep breath and hold it for five seconds, then exhale through your mouth, releasing all the tension in your hands and arms.
- Once you release the tension, press your arms down against the surface they are resting on and repeat the above sequence.
- Shrug your shoulders toward your head and hold them there for five to ten seconds. Take a deep breath and hold it for five seconds, then exhale through your mouth, releasing the tension in your shoulders.
- Tense the muscles in your face: wrinkle your forehead, clench your jaw, and open your mouth wide. Hold each of these contractions for five to ten seconds. Take a deep breath and hold it for five seconds, then exhale through your mouth, releasing all the tension in your face.
- Tighten your stomach muscles for five to ten seconds. Take a deep breath and hold it for five seconds, then exhale through your mouth while releasing the tension in your stomach.
- Contract the muscles in your buttocks and hips and press your heels and legs against the surface you are resting upon. Hold for five to ten seconds. Take a deep breath and hold it for five seconds, then exhale through your mouth, releasing all the tension in the contracted muscles.

- Arch your back and hold for five to ten seconds. Take a deep breath and hold it for five seconds, then gently let your back fall toward the surface you are lying on as you exhale and release the tension.

- Focus on your toes: Curl them under, hold for five to ten seconds, then relax and curl them toward your knees. Hold for five to ten seconds. Take a deep breath and hold it for five seconds, then exhale through your mouth while releasing the tension in your toes.

- Now focus on your face and, in your mind, notice how soft and relaxed you feel, from your face to your shoulders, stomach, arms, hands, chest, hips, legs, and feet. Remain in this position, relaxed, for a few moments. Get up slowly when you are ready.

## PSYCHOTHERAPY

Psychotherapy can be a powerful complement to the depression treatment programs we've talked about thus far. Although I don't believe every person who is depressed needs psychotherapy, I do believe it can enhance recovery in many cases, especially among people whose depression is related to a psychological event, such as death of a spouse, divorce, or another type of loss or trauma. The severe stress associated with such events suppresses neurotransmitters and endorphins. Amino acid therapy, nutritional supplements, and other efforts can make significant headway in eliminating the depression experienced by these individuals, but the addition of psychotherapy can be the factor that helps people make a faster and more satisfying recovery.

## Nadine's Story

Nadine is an example of someone who benefited greatly from psychotherapy. After her husband died suddenly in an accident at the age of fifty-six, Nadine plunged into a deep depression. Her daughter Ruthann became increasingly worried about her mother, especially as she continued to lose weight and to have great difficulty sleeping. After Nadine refused to see a therapist, her daughter talked her into coming to see me six months after her father's death.

Nadine's state of chronic stress had taken its toll on her neurotransmitter and hormone levels, as well as her nutritional status, and we started an amino acid and hormone program, along with dietary changes. But I felt that Nadine was a good candidate for psychotherapy to enhance the therapies we had initiated. She continued to resist, and after she had been on the other treatments for several months and was experiencing some improvement, I again emphasized the advantages of psychotherapy. She agreed, and her progress from that point on was remarkable. After six biweekly sessions, her depression significantly faded, and she weaned herself from the therapist.

## Cognitive-Behavioral Therapy

Psychotherapy encompasses several different treatment techniques, all of which involve talking with a licensed mental health professional who can help patients work through life's stressors. One approach often used with people who have mild to moderate depression is cognitive-behavioral therapy, in which individuals learn to identify and change their self-perceptions and incorporate new behaviors into their lives that help them better cope. Repeatedly, studies indicate that cognitive-behavioral therapy is as effective as antidepressants in the treatment of depression.

One of the most recent examples was published in the April 2005 issue of *Archives of General Psychiatry*. University of Pennsylvania researchers compared the efficacy of various anti-depressants with cognitive therapy in 240 individuals who were moderately to severely depressed. The 120 patients in the medication group were given paroxetine or placebo for eight weeks, and for those who did not respond to paroxetine, lithium or desipramine was added. The sixty patients in the cognitive therapy group attended one to two fifty-minute sessions each week for sixteen weeks. Another sixty patients received placebo only.

After sixteen weeks of treatment, 58 percent of patients taking antidepressants and 58 percent of those receiving cognitive therapy had improved. Remission rates in these two groups were similar: 46 percent in the medication group and 40 percent in the therapy group. This finding led the researchers to say, "It appears that cognitive therapy can be as effective as medications, even among more severely depressed outpatients, at least when provided by experienced cognitive therapists." But what about staying power? Do the benefits of medication and cognitive therapy go on once these treatments stop?

Again, University of Pennsylvania researchers conducted a study among moderately to severely depressed adults. Patients who had responded to cognitive therapy in a previous trial stopped treatment, and their response was compared with that of patients who had responded previously to medication and who also stopped treatment. Twelve months later, researchers found that patients who had stopped cognitive therapy were significantly less likely to relapse (31 percent) than patients who had stopped their medications (76 percent), and no more likely to relapse than patients who had continued to take their medication (31 percent versus 47 percent). Thus this study shows us two things: The benefits of cognitive therapy extend beyond the end of therapy sessions, and cognitive therapy is as effective as having individuals continue taking their medication.

## MASSAGE

After just one massage session, Jessica was hooked. "If I had known before how wonderful a massage can be, I would have been getting at least one a week." She laughs when her husband raises his eyebrows and quickly reassures him. "A massage costs less than a therapist, whom I've stopped seeing. I'm sleeping better and I feel more positive about myself."

Although massage won't cure depression, it certainly can improve its symptoms. Jessica found this to be true when she added massage to her treatment program, which also included amino acid therapy and nutritional therapy. Touch is a power tool in the treatment of depressive symptoms. Massage stimulates the body to rid itself of toxins and to secrete certain chemicals and hormones that can enhance mood. Invariably everyone who undergoes massage reports that the experience relieves tension and stress and puts a positive spin on the rest of their life.

Much of the positive feedback about massage in the treatment of depression is anecdotal, but a few studies have demonstrated good reports as well. At Florida Atlantic University, for example, researchers used electroencephalography (EEG) to monitor the brain activity of thirty depressed adolescents and assess the effects of massage therapy and music therapy on right frontal activity in the brain, which is associated with depression and negative emotions. Sixteen teens received music therapy only, and fourteen had massage only. The EEG showed that both therapies had positive effects on right frontal activity in the depressed teens. In another study of depressed teen mothers, those who received massage or relaxation therapy for five weeks had less anxiety and recordable changes in behavioral and stress hormones, including a decrease in pulse, anxious behavior, and salivary and urinary cortisol levels.

Massage can be an enjoyable and effective addition to your treatment program. You may choose the services of a professional masseuse, or if you have a partner who is willing to learn basic massage techniques, there are some excellent books and videos that explain the technique, as well as community-based classes in many cities. Some people learn couples therapeutic massage, which is also offered in some cities. If you need help finding a qualified practitioner or learning materials, see the appendix.

## SLEEP

"Lots of times I feel so depressed all I want to do is sleep, but I can't," says Lorraine, a thirty-four-year-old insurance adjuster. "I toss and turn, I get up, raid the refrigerator, turn on the TV, then I take a sleeping pill and wake up exhausted when the alarm goes off."

Like many people who are depressed, Lorraine suffers with insomnia and sleep disturbances. Insomnia is one of the main symptoms of clinical depression; oversleeping occurs in only about 15 percent of depressed people, most of whom have manic depression (bipolar disorder).

## The Serotonin Connection

A main cause of sleep difficulties is a serotonin deficiency, which is also a primary reason why depressed people have insomnia or other sleep disturbances and why restoring serotonin levels to a healthy point can make sleep problems disappear. Serotonin is the only substance from which the brain can produce melatonin, a hormone that is responsible for regulating the sleep–wake cycle. Here's how it works.

Melatonin is produced from serotonin by the pineal gland, which is located deep within the brain. The pineal gland is very sensitive to light; as the sun gets lower in the sky and eventually sets, the transformation of serotonin into melatonin increases, but only if there is enough serotonin to produce it. If an insufficient amount of melatonin is made, sleep will not come easily or at all. If you have the symptoms of a serotonin deficiency, restoring those levels should solve your sleep problems as well. (See chapters 6 and 9 for more information about melatonin.)

If you are taking antidepressants or other medications, one or more of the drugs may be causing your sleep disturbances. Talk to your doctor or therapist about changing or stopping your medication. This will become easier to do once you are on amino acid therapy and other steps to treat your depression.

Getting adequate sleep goes a long way toward improving mood, energy level, coping ability, and mental functioning. Here are a few natural strategies for better sleep:

- **Restore serotonin and melatonin levels.** Serotonin levels can be restored by taking 5-HTP or tryptophan (see chapter 4). At the same time, you may take a melatonin supplement to stimulate the restoration process. Melatonin comes in 0.3 to 10 mg doses, but a good starting dose is 0.5 mg at bedtime. The dose can be increased, although too high a dose can cause morning grogginess. Melatonin should only be taken for about seven to ten days at a time, though there is no evidence of harm if people take it on a continuous basis. If you are taking amino acids to boost your serotonin levels, you should soon be producing your own melatonin and can stop the supplement.

- **Set up a sleep schedule.** Many people find it helps to establish a pattern of going to bed and getting up at the same time every day, even weekends and days off from work. Although it may not seem to work at first, the body gradually gets into a routine.

- **Relax before retiring.** It's impossible to go to sleep when you're trying to solve the world's problems in your head. They can wait until morning. Meditate, do slow stretches, take a warm bath, practice visualization, listen to soothing music, or watch an old movie on TV.

- **Establish bedtime traditions.** Did your parents read to you before you went to sleep? Give you warm milk? Let you take your stuffed animals to bed with you? Bedtime traditions are comforting at any age, so you might want to create a few of your own just for you.

- **Avoid alcohol, nicotine, and caffeine.** If you do indulge at all, avoid use from midafternoon onward. Alcohol is a depressant (nicotine and caffeine are stimulants), which can help you fall asleep, but you will likely wake up in the middle of the night and be unable to fall back asleep.

- **Make your sleep environment comfortable.** Feeling too hot or too cold, excessive light, or sleeping on an uncomfortable mattress are common but correctable complaints.
- **Get some exercise.** The best times to exercise are during the day up to early evening, but not within three or four hours of bedtime; the stimulation may make it harder to fall asleep.
- **Go to bed "just right."** Going to bed hungry can make you wake up much earlier than you'd like, while going to bed with a full stomach can be uncomfortable. If you need a snack before bedtime, make it a light one, but one containing some protein, such as some nuts or seeds or a glass of organic milk or a piece of organic cheese.

## NURTURING FAMILY AND OTHER MEANINGFUL RELATIONSHIPS

Although throughout this book, I have emphasized many topics that are not usually found in books about depression, I want to emphasize here that loving family and other meaningful relationships are extremely important in preventing and treating depression. As I have tried to stress throughout the book, how you feel is a function of many different variables, and they all interrelate with one another. When one variable is out of balance, it may have disastrous effects on other variables and the whole system in general. So all of the topics we've discussed can contribute to impaired loving relationships, and correcting imbalances may pave the way for repairing and nurturing relationships with problems. Frequently, imbalances in a spouse or partner can also play a role in the impaired relationship. Whenever possible these should be addressed.

One approach to improving relationships of all kinds is

to focus on improved communication. I have been particularly impressed by the program outlined by Harville Hendrix, PhD, in his book *Getting the Love You Want: A Guide for Couples*. This is an excellent self-help book, but since it was published, he has trained many therapists in his techniques of Imago Therapy. Trained therapists for couples are available in many areas of the United States, and qualified therapists can be found at various websites.

## PERSONAL GROWTH

"I admit I was resistant at first," says Connie, a fifty-year-old part-time pastry chef at a five-star resort. "My therapist recommended I do volunteer work because she said it would get me 'out of my head.' Yet after work all I wanted to do was go home and hibernate; I was always so depressed. Then my sister volunteered both of us to walk and play with the dogs at an animal shelter on the weekend because she knows I love dogs. It didn't take long before I was hooked. Now I go once or twice during the week after work and on weekends. It's great working with the dogs. I can't remember the last time I've looked forward to something so much. I feel like I'm doing something important."

Depression is a very isolating, lonely state of being. One way to break out of the "black hole," as some patients call it, is to reach out and connect with someone or something that is meaningful—something that gives you direction, a sense of purpose, a reason to get out of bed in the morning, or a feeling of being in tune with others and with the world. Connie found her reason by working with abandoned and neglected dogs, but there are thousands of things you can do to break through the isolating and self-defeating cloak of depression. There's even convincing evidence that it works.

## Religious and Spiritual Connections

Some researchers have set out to scientifically document what impact a person's relationship with God, a higher power, nature, or another sacred or spiritual ideal has on depression and mood. One of the first articles to tackle that idea was published in 1998 in the *American Journal of Psychiatry*. Among the depressed elderly individuals studied, those with a strong religious faith were better able to cope with life changes and to recover from depression. Going to church and participating in religious activities, such as Bible or prayer study, however, were not factors.

In other studies, it's been shown that there's a decreased rate of depression and suicide among people who participate in spiritual activities. Research also shows that higher spirituality scores correlate with fewer symptoms of depression, as in a Yale University study in which 122 people participated. The experts found that among depressed and nondepressed individuals, those in the latter category were significantly more likely to believe in a higher power, have a relationship with a higher power, and believe in prayer.

Jon Kabat-Zinn, PhD, author of *Wherever You Go, There You Are* and founder and director of the Stress Reduction Clinic at the University of Massachusetts Medical Center, suggests that people make an effort to be mindful of their environment; to find purpose, meaning, and beauty in every experience and through all their senses. Dr. Kabat-Zinn practices and teaches a form of meditation called mindfulness that, he says, helps people "in times of great stress or pain . . . [because] they know how to go to their breathing, to use it to calm down and broaden the field of perception, so that they can see with a larger perspective."

## Making Other Connections

Connecting with something meaningful or sacred can take many forms. Any connection an individual makes is his or her own; even if two people choose journaling to express their feelings, the product of their work will be unique to each.

• **Turn to the arts.** Expressing yourself through art, be it painting, drawing, sculpting, music, or dance, can be very therapeutic for many people suffering with depression. Some people discover talents they never knew they possessed; others simply find joy in the creative process. Art therapy is available at various facilities. Though we do not do this at the Schachter Center, we believe it is worthwhile for some people.

• **Write it down.** Journaling, writing poetry or stories, or composing letters can provide a tangible way to connect with and express your feelings, resolve conflicts, and reach out to others. You don't need to share what you write, however. Daria began writing poetry during her treatment for depression, and says it is a tremendous release. But she's not ready to share her work with the world. "The poems are too personal, too bleak right now," she says. "But I really enjoy writing them and how I feel when I'm done, like I've accomplished something, like I'm okay with the world."

• **Reach out to nature.** Distancing yourself from the hurry-day world and allowing yourself to experience nature firsthand can be a great source of comfort. Natural settings are also conducive to meditation, journaling, and other contemplative activities.

• **Join a support group.** "One of the worst things about being depressed is that you feel so alone," says Lynette, a forty-year-old hairdresser and single mom who had a very difficult time coping with the death of her fourteen-year-old daughter in a car accident. "For the first six months after Tiffany died, I couldn't cope with daily life. My friends and family tried to help, but I didn't think they could really understand what I was going through. Then my best friend found a support group for parents who had lost a child, and she literally drove me to the front door of the meeting. Being with those parents was one of the saddest yet most uplifting things I've ever done. I found love, understanding, and courage, and a way out of my depression." Ask your doctor or local hospital about area support groups. The appendix lists some resources for both live and on-line support groups.

• **Learn something new.** Have you always wanted to learn Italian cooking? Photography? Tai chi? Sign language? Swimming? Learning something new is like starting a whole new chapter in your life, a chapter that will include your feeling better about yourself.

• **Volunteer.** Choose a cause that is meaningful to you, such as fighting breast cancer, spaying and neutering pets, literacy, or preserving forests. Contact a local nonprofit organization that supports the cause of your choice or visit your local library for a list of nonprofits or social service groups in your area.

## THE BOTTOM LINE

You may dramatically improve your recovery from depression if you make a few lifestyle changes, especially if they are done along with amino acid therapy and other treatments discussed throughout this book. In this chapter, you've seen how lifestyle activities can have a direct impact on substances in the body that are intimately associated with mood. Mind–body works together as a whole, in illness and in health, and is naturally geared toward balance. This fact is all the more reason why depression and other mood disorders should be treated with natural means whenever possible—and what better way to accomplish this than to make lifestyle choices that heal?

## Chapter 11

# Energy Medicine

When you are depressed, your entire body is in a state of imbalance—physically, emotionally, mentally, and spiritually. Thus, it makes sense to take steps to bring these facets back into harmony. Energy medicine can be instrumental in helping to correct imbalances in the body that contribute to a depressed mood.

In this chapter, we step back from the "hard-core" biochemical approaches to treatment of depression—amino acid therapy, diet, nutritional supplements, and herbs—and step into the realm of bioenergy, which includes, among other things, such healing techniques as acupuncture, homeopathy, and Reiki. These three bioenergy techniques in particular have proved helpful for many of the patients at the Schachter Center. I also encourage you to explore forms of energy medicine not covered in this chapter and offer some resources in the suggested reading list.

## BODY AS ENERGY

Eastern and other nontraditional healing traditions are curious phenomena for many people in the United States, even as they are becoming accepted by some mainstream medical professionals. This is especially true as researchers conduct studies that explore these therapies and report on their ability, in many cases, to provide effective, safe relief from depression and other mood disorders.

Among nontraditional healing methods is energy medicine, the definition of which shifts, based on the type of practitioner with whom you speak. Generally, however, energy medicine is a practice in which a trained individual works with the body's energy field to improve physical, emotional, mental, and/or spiritual health. This definition embraces many different practices, ranging from acupuncture to homeopathy to therapeutic touch to prayer circles.

Before you dismiss energy medicine as hocus-pocus or a waste of time, let me assure you that energy therapies have a firm scientific basis in an area of physics called quantum electrodynamics, or QED. Robert E. Connolly, DSc, LAc, an expert in biofeedback acupuncture, energetic rebalancing, and detoxification, has worked at the Schachter Center for the past seventeen years. He explains that, within only the last few decades, scientists have become increasingly aware that all biochemical processes in the body are driven by subatomic energy fields, and that the body's cells communicate with one another using electromagnetic signals. You've already learned that biochemical balance is essential for optimal health, and now we add one more element to the picture: electromagnetic balance—clear communication among cells. In fact, since biochemical and bioenergetic processes operate at the same time, it's critical that these processes be in balance with each other.

I believe energy medicine therapies can be very beneficial in establishing a balance between the biochemical and bioenergetic processes. Because there are many different energy medicine approaches, I'll limit this discussion to those that have demonstrated the most effectiveness in the treatment of mood disorders. This is not to say that any I haven't included may not be helpful to you.

## ACUPUNCTURE

The addition of acupuncture to a treatment plan for depression has been quite rewarding for some of my patients. Traditionally, this ancient holistic healing technique, rooted in traditional Chinese medicine, has been used to prevent disease and illness, but it also is effective in the treatment of pain and other conditions, including depression.

### How It Works

Acupuncture involves the insertion of fine needles along various points in the body (meridians) that have been identified as being associated with different organs and symptoms. According to traditional Chinese medicine, the purpose of inserting these needles is to stimulate the body's flow of energy, referred to as *qi* or *chi*. Research indicates that stimulating such points causes the release of endorphins, and too little endorphin activity, as I've already explained, is associated with depression.

Some practitioners use needles through which they pass a very mild electrical current. Known as electroacupuncture, both it and conventional acupuncture have proven effective in the treatment of depression and related symptoms.

While the idea of being stuck with needles is disconcerting to some people, others, like Maureen, put skepticism aside and are ready for the experience. In her case, acupuncture, applied kinesiology (a system that utilizes acupuncture knowledge to obtain information about the patient) with muscle testing, the use of homeopathic remedies (different from the classical homeopathy described on page 293), and a variety of other techniques were used to bring her back to a healthy state.

Maureen, a married homemaker in her early forties with two children, came to see our acupuncturist Bob Connolly. She had complained of chronic fatigue, headaches, weight gain, and depression for more than five years. Over the past two years, however, she had become worse, saying that she was very negative toward the world in general and often avoided social activities. "Everything seems like too much effort," she said. "I'm just not interested in things anymore." This lack of interest extended to a loss of sex drive, but she claimed she didn't care about that specific problem.

Her diet was fairly good except she said she needed coffee each morning to get started, and about six months before she sought treatment she had begun to drink a few bottles of high-fat, high-sugar coffee drinks daily. Soon after she started those drinks she began to gain weight, but she said she felt "an intense desire" to continue drinking them. She believed she has some food allergies to wheat and dairy in particular.

An acupuncture examination revealed excessive activity in the liver meridian and deficient activity in the kidney meridian, which is associated with adrenal stress or fatigue from a conventional medical perspective, as well as indications of disturbances in the endocrine system. Kinesiology indicated multiple food sensitivities, none of them severe. She was prescribed once-weekly acupuncture sessions that mainly treated the liver excess, kidney weakness, and endocrine system. She was also treated with an electronic acupuncture device that scanned for disturbances and made adjustments electronically without needles.

Maureen also had dental problems that she chose not to address, even though we strongly urged her to see a dentist. Based on the results of muscle testing against her liver and teeth, she was given the homeopathic remedy hypericum daily for two months and then nux vomica for two weeks. Nutritional supplementation was kept to a minimum because Maureen usually felt worse after taking supplements. We were able to give her minimal supplementation when muscle testing indicated she could tolerate it, and as a result she significantly reduced her use of coffee and sugar.

Over a three-month period, her depression gradually lifted, her energy level increased substantially, she lost weight, and her headaches nearly disappeared. She is now very socially active, has a leadership role in her community, and feels she is at a point in her life where she can maximize her potential.

## Acupuncture and Depression

Many of the studies conducted to examine the use of acupuncture in depression have been done with women. In several such studies done since the turn of the millennium, researchers found that acupuncture appears to be effective as the sole therapy for major depression and as a promising treatment for depression associated with pregnancy.

These studies had precedents. In 1998, the first randomized, controlled, double-blind study of acupuncture's effectiveness for depression reported in Western scientific literature found that among thirty-eight women diagnosed with mild to moderate depression, 70 percent of them experienced at least a 50 percent reduction of depressive symptoms after twelve acupuncture sessions. These results are comparable to the success rates of psychotherapy and medication. In another study, forty-three patients with minor depression and thirteen with general anxiety disorders were treated with either acupuncture or placebo acupuncture (in which techniques are used that are not intended to stimulate known acupuncture points for depression). After ten sessions, patients with depression or anxiety who had true acupuncture were significantly better and reported a "remarkable reduction in anxiety symptoms" compared with patients who received placebo.

Acupuncture can be an effective complement to your depression treatment program. To help you find a competent acupuncture practitioner, please see the appendix.

## HOMEOPATHY

Few health-care practitioners consider homeopathy when they think about treating depression, but I find that it can be a very helpful complementary therapy for some patients. Homeopathic remedies can shift a person's energetic balance and factors that have an impact on that balance—such as emotional scars that may have formed from emotional trauma—and provide dramatic results.

## How It Works

Homeopathy is based on two basic principles: the Law of Similars and potentization. If you've ever gotten a flu shot or another type of vaccination, you've experienced how the Law of Similars works. Basically, the law states that exposure to a substance that can cause certain symptoms in a healthy person can, when given in minute amounts, stimulate the body to relieve similar symptoms in an ailing individual.

For example, if you've ever chopped an onion, you've likely experienced watery, burning eyes, sneezing, a runny nose, and an irritated throat. In homeopathy, a remedy called allium cepa, made of red onion, is used to help overcome symptoms of a cold or allergy—symptoms like those just named.

The remedy, like other homeopathic remedies, comes in the form of a tiny pill or granules that have been carefully prepared through a process called potentization. Potentization involves taking a specific substance, such as red onion, dissolving it in solution, and then diluting it with a solvent. It is then diluted repeatedly. After each dilution, the remedy is vigorously shaken (called succussion). During this process of potentization, it is believed that energy is transferred from the original substance to the diluent or water molecules. Interestingly, the more dilute the remedy, the stronger its healing properties. When someone takes a remedy, it transfers its energy to the person, initiating a healing response.

The potency of a remedy is related to the number of times it has been diluted and succussed. Each homeopathic remedy is associated with a number and a letter. The number refers to how many times the remedy had been diluted, while the letter refers to the concentration of each dilution. The corresponding letters for each concentration are as follows: X is 1:10; C is 1:100, and M is 1:1,000. So, for example, a 12X remedy has been diluted twelve times, each time with a concentration of 1 part of the active ingredient with 9 parts of the diluent (often water). A 200C potency has been diluted two hundred times, each with a concentration of 1 part remedy to 99 parts diluent. Using these methods, some potencies contain no molecules of the original substance, but only the transferred energy. This diluted homeopathic remedy can then be given either as a liquid or as sugar pellets that are infused with the homeopathic liquid remedy.

Homeopathy has its share of skeptics, especially among conventional physicians. However, a slowly growing number of formal studies published in medical journals show that homeopathic remedies can be more effective than placebo when treating certain conditions. It's been theorized that the ability of homeopathic remedies to heal is associated with the energy change that occurs during potentization, which in turn stimulates a person's body to better cope with whatever stressors are causing the illness. Further studies may help us learn whether this or other forces are at work in homeopathy.

## Classical Homeopathy and Depression

Some homeopathic remedies have demonstrated the ability to help individuals who are living with depression and associated symptoms. However, homeopathic treatment of depression requires the skill of a well-trained classical homeopath and should not be undertaken by reading a book or requesting treatment from someone who does not know the field very well. A classical homeopath must take a detailed homeopathic history that emphasizes the particular individuality of a person and his or her symptoms. Then, depending upon the nature of the symptoms, their intensity, peculiar characteristics related to the symptoms, and other factors, the classical homeopath matches the patient with a particular remedy and administers it. Here are some of the remedies used by a classical homeopath:

• **Arsenicum album.** This remedy is best for individuals who are susceptible to depression and who also suffer from anxiety (especially about health matters) and insecurity. These people tend to be perfectionists and are very negative. They also tend to feel chilly much of the time and may suffer from severe phobias.

• **Aurum metallicum.** This remedy frequently works for people who have deep depression with thoughts of suicide. Such patients who wish to be treated homeopathically must seek help from a very experienced classical homeopath who will need to determine whether treatment outside a hospital is reasonably safe. The patient should probably also be evaluated by a psychiatrist trained to evaluate the suicide risk to determine if hospitalization is necessary.

• **Calcarea carbonica.** Hardworking, dependable people who become overwhelmed from too much work, stress, or physical illness may be helped by this remedy. Their depression may be accompanied by anxiety, confusion, self-pity, and a dread of disaster. People who benefit from calcarea often feel sluggish and chilly.

• **Causticum.** Those who are experiencing loss or grief may benefit from this remedy. Characteristics of those who may be helped include frequent crying, forgetfulness, a strong sense of injustice, and anger toward the world.

- **Ignatia.** People who benefit from this remedy usually are those whose depression is the result of grief or emotional trauma; it is characterized by rapid mood changes. Frequent sighing and sensations of a lump in the throat are common among people helped by this remedy.

- **Kali phosphoricum.** This remedy is most helpful for individuals whose depression is the result of overwork and who are experiencing mental fatigue.

- **Natrum muriaticum.** If you don't want to reveal your emotions and typically hold your feelings inside, this homeopathic remedy may help you. Those who benefit from natrum muriaticum often become aggravated when people try to console them, and they have an aversion to sunlight and a strong craving for salt.

- **Pulsatilla.** Works best in people who burst into tears at little or no provocation. Often they seek constant comfort and are very sensitive. Their depressive symptoms worsen in warm environments, and for women, they are worse around their menstrual cycle or menopause.

- **Sepia.** This remedy is for women who feel indifferent to their families and who have a low sex drive and suffer from fatigue and irritability. They feel worse when consoled and better when they exercise. Their depression is often associated with hormone imbalances.

- **Staphysagria.** Those who benefit from this remedy are people with suppressed emotions that contribute to their depression. Such individuals are usually quiet. Headache and insomnia are common symptoms that accompany their low mood.

**Taking Homeopathic Remedies**

Homeopathic remedies have a reputation for being safe and nontoxic, but that does not mean they should be used indiscriminately. In fact, choosing the optimal remedies for an individual is an art, as they must be selected to match a person's current health condition and how he or she uniquely responds to the environment. Choosing an inappropriate remedy will not result in harm, but it will offer little or no benefit. Although many people are tempted to forgo a professional's advice when using homeopathic remedies, I recommend you work with a knowledgeable classical homeopath if you want to try homeopathy. Here are a few reasons why:

- You may have serious medical issues other than your depression that need to be evaluated and treated professionally.
- Sometimes symptoms become worse temporarily when you first take a homeopathic remedy, even when the remedy is correctly selected. However, only an experienced professional can distinguish between such transient aggravation of symptoms and a medical condition that is progressing.
- People who self-treat are sometimes tempted to take too many doses or switch to another remedy before giving the current remedy sufficient time. A professional can help you make informed decisions about dosing.
- A homeopath can conduct the necessary in-depth interview and history that will allow him or her to identify the remedy that best fits your characteristic symptoms and considers your physical, emotional, and mental nature.

Remedies are typically taken as follows: The homeopath administers or instructs the patient to take one dose and wait for a response, usually about four or five weeks. If symptoms improve, then the treatment is not repeated; rather, the remedy is allowed to continue to work. If there is no improvement, the homeopath obtains more information and then decides to either repeat the remedy, give it at a higher potency, or change the remedy altogether. Some people believe that if they get a positive response after taking a homeopathic remedy, they should take another one immediately, mistakenly thinking that if one dose is good, two or more will be better. However, taking unnecessary doses can actually slow down or interfere with a remedy's action. The frequency of dosing is variable and depends on the individual and his or her condition and response.

Sometimes the results of classic homeopathy can be dramatic and almost miraculous. The following story was related to me by Sue Anello, a classical homeopath who has consulted at the Schachter Center.

Mary, a thirty-year-old mother, appeared for homeopathic treatment six months after her first baby was born. She said that she felt that she couldn't be happy. She described herself as a "total bitch" to her husband and said nothing satisfied her anymore. Her baby, she said, was whiny and cried a lot, especially at night.

She also reported that her shoulders hurt all the time, and that she felt "too lousy" to exercise. In the past, she had found that vigorous exercise helped her to feel better, especially when she broke into a sweat. Now, however, "I don't want to get out of bed," she said. "I'm never rested, even if I go to bed at nine thirty. I hate to hear the baby cry. I'm tense and angry and keep asking, *Why, why?* I thought I'd be overjoyed to be a mother."

She said she was mourning the loss of her old life and just wanted to scream at the baby. She hated her husband and felt he just didn't understand her, and often she found herself yelling at him or giving him the silent treatment. She craved chocolate, salty foods, and deli meats, was worse in the late afternoon, and felt warm all the time even though she had always tended to feel chilled.

Mary was given one dose of the homeopathic remedy sepia 1M and told to return for follow-up one month later. At that visit, she reported that on her way home the day she was given sepia, "The sun came out as I drove over the bridge." She had felt better within minutes of taking the remedy. The rest of the appointment she talked about her excitement over new projects in her life. She has since had a second baby with no recurrence of depression.

Not all cases result in this kind of dramatic and rapid response. Sometimes, results may take quite a bit longer. But a skilled classical homeopath can often do wonders for a depressed patient.

If you need help finding a qualified homeopath, including medical homeopaths (those who also have an MD license), see the appendix.

## REIKI

Reiki is a form of energy medicine in which healing energy is channeled through a practitioner into the individual receiving the treatment. The name of this self-healing approach comes from the Japanese *rei*, which means "universal," and *ki*, which means "energy." Practitioners of Reiki believe that when *ki* (also referred to as *qi* or *chi*) is blocked, depression and illness can develop. Reiki facilitates the removal of blocked energy, helps eliminate toxins from the body, and helps individuals cope with depression and anxiety.

Heart transplant patients at Yale–New Haven Medical Center in Connecticut have been enjoying the benefits of Reiki for several years. At this world-class facility, all new patients in the coronary care unit are offered Reiki, as well as other nontraditional treatments, along with conventional care.

It's true that evidence of Reiki's ability to relieve depression is primarily anecdotal, but at least one study has been published. Adina Goldman Shore, PhD, studied the long-term effects of Reiki on depression and stress in forty-five individuals over a one-year period. The volunteers were assigned to one of three groups: hands-on Reiki, long-distance Reiki, or placebo (sham long-distance Reiki sessions). Each participant received one ninety-minute session weekly for six weeks. Three tests designed to measure stress and depression were administered both before and after the treatment period.

While participants in the two treatment groups experienced improvement in depression and stress, those in the placebo group did not. One year after the six sessions, the three tests were readministered, and individuals in the placebo group were given actual Reiki treatments and retested after the sessions. This time the volunteers reported relief from depression and stress.

Some researchers believe that the deep relaxation people experience with Reiki stimulates the release of endorphins. Evelyn, a forty-four-year-old hairdresser who has had several Reiki sessions, sums it up by saying, "I really don't know how it works, but it does. I feel more aware of my surroundings, more focused, and much less stress. I'm not going to argue with success."

## How It Works

While Reiki should not be used as a substitute for other treatments for depression, it has been an effective complementary approach for many of my patients. A typical Reiki session lasts sixty to ninety minutes, but shorter sessions can be arranged. During a treatment, you lie fully clothed on a comfortable table in a room where there may be lighted candles or soothing music playing in the background. The Reiki practitioner will likely move his or her hands a few inches above your entire body, "scanning" for energy blockages. Practitioners reportedly can identify such blockages when they feel tingling or a warm sensation in their hands. Once problem areas have been identified, the practitioner will gently keep his or her hands over those spots, channeling energy into the area for three to five minutes (or longer if the area is especially blocked).

At the Schachter Center, one of our staff members, Sandra Davis, is a master Reiki practitioner who works with some of our patients.

If you are interested in locating a Reiki practitioner, talk to your health-care provider for recommendations, or see the appendix for assistance.


## THE BOTTOM LINE

At the most basic level, you are a mass of bioenergy, moving among other forms of energy and interacting with them at varying levels. When your bioenergy is disturbed by stress and illness, it makes sense to restore it to a harmonious state. Bioenergy medicine provides you with natural, effective ways to help achieve balance. The methods discussed in this chapter are meant to complement other treatments for depression explained elsewhere in this volume.

# Chapter 12

—— ❦ ——

# Psychotropic Drugs: What's the Story?

Antidepressants and other mind-altering drugs (psychotropics) are the first options most people think of when treatment of depression is discussed, but many practitioners and most consumers are not aware of their limitations. My goal in this chapter is to give you a glimpse of the story behind the drugs used to treat depression and mood disorders. Here I summarize some of the controversies as well as important facts about available drugs to treat depression and related conditions with emphasis on some of the problems, adverse effects, and drug interactions that may occur. I believe consumers need to be aware of these issues, because frequently this information is not readily available.

Dr. Allen Roses, a world-renowned geneticist and the current vice president of genetics at GlaxoSmithKline, stated at a December 2003 scientific meeting, "Fewer than half of the patients prescribed some of the most expensive drugs actually derive any benefit from them." This view of the limits of pharmaceuticals contrasts sharply with the standard view of the majority of physicians that most drugs are potent, safe, effective, and scientific. On the other hand, conventional medicine views nutraceuticals (biological substances such as vitamin, mineral, and amino acid supplements) as being weak, dangerous, ineffective, unproven, and substances to avoid. The reality, according to Paul Hardy, MD, a psychiatrist who has held faculty positions in neurology and psychiatry at Tufts University School of Medicine and Harvard Medical School, is that "pharmaceuticals depend upon proper nutrition for optimal action. Moreover, pharmaceuticals are extremely dependent on proper nutrition for their inactivation and removal from the body." He further points out that conventional physicians, including psychiatrists, are highly biased against nutritional, orthomolecular, or complementary approaches.

The focus at the Schachter Center is to use pharmaceuticals responsibly along with nutraceuticals and other available modalities with the goal of eventually getting people to stop taking medications whenever possible, because we simply do not know all the long-term adverse effects of taking a substance that is foreign to the body. Whenever we can clear away depression and encourage health without the use of drugs, we do this.

## THE TROUBLE WITH PSYCHOTROPIC MEDICATIONS

The trouble with psychotropic medications goes deeper than the fact that they may be ineffective in the treatment of depression and other mood-related disorders. They may also have significant adverse effects. Here are some of the considerations that may relate both to possible lack of effectiveness and to possible adverse side effects.

## How Drug Studies Are Conducted

Part of the problem with psychotropic drugs can be attributed to how they are tested before they are brought to market. In most cases, studies are conducted in relevant patient groups for eight to nine weeks at most, which frequently is not enough time for some side effects to become evident. Most notably, systemic reactions (those that affect the whole body) may take many months to develop, or subtle effects on the brain such as memory problems may not become apparent for some time. Often, patients and doctors don't make a connection between use of the medication and the development of new symptoms (such as impaired memory), since the patient has been on the medication for some time before the new symptoms develop. The causal relationship may not be seen until after the person has stopped the medication and notices that the symptom subsides or after the symptom subsides and reappears after medication use resumes.

Another problem is in how the studies are structured. For example, if you don't specifically ask someone if he or she has noticed any change in sex drive since starting a drug, you won't know if there has been a change. Some people may not attribute a side effect to a drug, especially when it concerns sensitive issues such as sexual performance or bladder control. If a study isn't designed to ask the right questions, or if the participants are somehow made to feel uncomfortable when answering sensitive questions, the researchers are going to get reports of a much lower incidence of some adverse reactions.

## The Problem with Drug Interactions

Because so many people take more than one medication—prescription and/or over the counter—and are using nutritional supplements and herbal remedies, a special concern is drug interactions. Do you know how your body will respond, for example, if you take an over-the-counter cough suppressant that contains dextromethorphan while also taking the antidepressant paroxetine (Paxil)? This may seem like a harmless thing to do; indeed, many people think that over-the-counter drugs are safer than prescription drugs. However, it's important to remember that *any* drug may interact negatively with another drug, herbal remedies, and even nutrients. In the case of dextromethorphan and paroxetine, this mixture may lead to serotonin syndrome, a condition triggered by increased stimulation of serotonin and characterized by fever, nausea, diarrhea, high blood pressure, tremor, seizures, confusion, insomnia, and headache, among others.

Unfortunately, when a new drug is brought to market, very little is known about how it will interact with other medications, because generally *no studies are done involving the new drug combined with other drugs already on the market.* Pharmaceutical companies can wait for doctors and patients to report adverse drug reactions, but they are relying on reports that are coming in *after the drug has been approved by the Food and Drug Administration.* They can also depend on what's been reported about drug interactions in the past with drugs that are similar to the one just released to the public. Thus Effexor (venlafaxine), an antidepressant that was released after paroxetine and is similar to it (both are selective serotonin reuptake inhibitors, although Effexor is also a norepinephrine reuptake inhibitor), has also been shown to cause serotonin syndrome if taken along with dextromethorphan.

## Drug Marketing Incentives

Another problem related to the prescription of antidepressants and other psychotropic medications is how psychiatrists and other health-care practitioners are often manipulated by pharmaceutical companies to prescribe drugs for their patients. Physicians are provided with free samples, free seminars that are supposed to be free from commercial bias (but actually aren't), as well as "incentives," such as expensive dinners and free trips to conferences at exotic locations, to "encourage" them to prescribe the drugs a specific pharmaceutical company is selling. Studies show that physicians are much more likely to prescribe drugs for which they have been given free samples. Other research shows that physicians' use of two drugs before and after they were sent on a free trip to learn more about the medications increased more than threefold while their use of other drugs remained unchanged. Pharmaceutical companies often ask psychiatrists to conduct drug studies, for which they are paid, and then to lecture about the drug at conferences, subtly pushing their products. These companies spend about $15 billion per year, or nearly $10,000 per physician, to influence drug-prescribing habits.

## Advertising Glitz

Gone are the days when the drug companies spent all their advertising budget on convincing doctors to prescribe their products. In recent years, pharmaceutical companies have spent billions advertising their products directly to consumers. Such direct-to-consumer ads are designed to make an emotional impact and are largely directed at women, even when the drug is for men. In 2000, drug companies spent $2.5 billion in direct-to-consumer advertising, and nearly 90 percent of consumers learn about brand-name drugs through manufacturers' ads, with 89 percent of them appearing on TV.

Are manufacturers being responsible advertisers? In August 2002, *Red Flags Weekly* reported that despite the fact that 25 percent of Prozac users experienced side effects, Eli Lilly spent $15 million to advertise the drug directly to the public to increase patient demand for it from their doctors. According to an FDA physicians' survey, only 40 percent of doctors believe their patients understand very well or somewhat well the possible risks and negative effects of an advertised drug from the direct-to-consumer ad alone. This is not surprising. Spend a few hours watching television and you will likely see at least half a dozen ads for prescription drugs, depicting pleasant scenes, smiling actors, and a list of side effects glossed over so you don't realize you've heard them.

Are manufacturers intentionally downplaying the negatives of their products? I believe they would prefer to see it as emphasizing the positives rather than highlighting the negatives. In any case, a January 2004 report from the Committee on Government Reform noted that the FDA's *enforcement* of prescription drug ad regulations continued to decline in 2003, and that misleading or false ads were running for months before they were cited. This is just another example of why you should be wary of any drugs on the market.

## Drug Study Cover-Ups?

Another problem with drug studies is that some pharmaceutical companies have been suppressing negative findings, giving the public a false view of the safety and effectiveness of their drugs. A case in point is the June 2004 lawsuit brought by New York Attorney General Eliot Spitzer against GlaxoSmithKline (GSK), which makes Paxil. The lawsuit alleged that GSK committed fraud by intentionally withholding negative study results and misrepresenting data concerning the use of the drug in children and adolescents. Withholding this information, said Spitzer, "impaired doctors' ability to make the appropriate prescribing decision for their patients and may have jeopardized their health and safety." Although Paxil had not been approved by the FDA for treatment of depression in children, health-care practitioners have professional discretion to prescribe it for "off-label" use, discretion many physicians have utilized.

Specifically, of the five or more studies GSK conducted on the use of Paxil in children and adolescents, it published and distributed the results of only one, and that one showed mixed effectiveness. The lawsuit claimed that the company suppressed the negative results of the other studies, including information suggesting that the drug may cause an increased risk of suicidal thinking and behavior. To make matters worse, GSK sales representatives portrayed the drug as having "remarkable efficacy and safety" when used in depressed adolescents. In fact, however, GSK submitted documents to the FDA and similar organizations in Europe and England in which it admitted that its studies "all failed to separate [Paxil] from placebo overall and so do not provide strong evidence of efficacy in this indication."

The lawsuit was settled in August 2004, and one week later, GlaxoSmithKline agreed to post the results of its clinical trials since 2000 online. Another pharmaceutical company, Eli Lilly, made plans to create a database as well. At the same time, the American Medical Association asked federal authorities to create a national database where drug companies would be required to post their trial results for public inspection.

There are critics of drug studies from within the psychiatric community as well. Soon after Alex Braiman, MD, a practicing psychiatrist, was awarded a fifty-year "distinguished fellow award" from the American Psychiatric Association in May 2004, he wrote a letter to *Psychiatric News* in which he said, "It is ironic that we are witnessing serious challenges to the scientific integrity of studies supporting the FDA approval of the SSRI class of antidepressants at a time when an unsilent majority of us go along with the pretense that this is evidence-based psychiatry."

None of this is to say that all pharmaceutical companies are suppressing negative study results or that they are intentionally manipulating data to present a more favorable image of their products. However, those companies that may be doing so may find that the public's growing insistence for the truth about research results makes such dealings impossible, which would be a clear victory for consumers.

## PHARMACEUTICALS VERSUS NUTRACEUTICALS

In her book *The Truth about Drug Companies: How They Deceive Us and What to Do About It*, Marcia Angell, MD, the former editor in chief of the *New England Journal of Medicine*, stated, "Drug companies have enormous influence over what doctors are taught about drugs and what they prescribe." She went on to say that "nutraceuticals [such as vitamins, herbs, amino acids] are not patentable and therefore less commercially profitable."

The very strong negative opinions about alternative medicine by conventional medicine practitioners are well reflected in a 1998 editorial in the *New England Journal of Medicine* by this same Dr. Angell and Dr. Kassirer. Along with characterizing alternative medicine as running "the risks of untested and unregulated remedies," they stated:

- "With the increased interest in alternative medicine, we see a reversion to irrational approaches to medical practice."
- "Some people may embrace alternative medicine exclusively, putting themselves in great danger."
- "It is time for the scientific community to stop giving alternative medicine a free ride. There cannot be two kinds of medicine . . . there is only medicine that has been adequately tested."

The problem with viewing conventional medicine as adequately tested and alternative medicine as not is that it takes several hundred million dollars to conduct the years of premarketing research and animal studies required to get a drug approved by the FDA, and only wealthy pharmaceutical companies have the means to do this kind of testing. These companies are not going to use their resources to research unpatentable drugs. Hence, nutraceuticals will never be researched to the satisfaction of physicians like Drs. Angell and Kassirer.

This bias against nutritional approaches and for the use of conventional medicine has not always been the case. Hippocrates said, "Let food be your medicine and . . . medicine be your food." Sir William Osler (1849–1919), one of the great leaders of modern medicine, said, "One of the first duties of the physician is to educate the masses not to take medicine," and "The desire to take medicine is perhaps the greatest feature which distinguishes man from animals."

Although I am willing to use medications, I prefer to seek the root of the problem, which involves looking at how a person's genetic makeup or characteristics can interact with important environmental factors to cause problems. I then look to correct that problem using nutraceuticals whenever possible (along with approaches discussed in this book), saving pharmaceuticals as the last resort.

## Psychotropics and Neurotransmitters

When the first antidepressants hit the market in the late 1950s, they paved the way for a steady stream of other drugs that affect mood, including antianxiety, mood-stabilizing, and antipsychotic medications. In general, psychotropic drugs either alter the receptors of neurotransmitters or increase the presence of neurotransmitters in the synapse, thereby increasing some of their effects or altering responses in some other way. What they don't do is increase neurotransmitter production. For this function, natural precursors and not synthetic medications are necessary. Therefore, for psychotropic drugs to work effectively, sufficient neurotransmitters must be present, because:

- Psychotropic drugs cannot increase the production of neurotransmitters.
- They do not work properly unless an individual already has an adequate supply of neurotransmitters.
- Psychotropic drugs sometimes stop working when neurotransmitter levels fall, sometimes due in part to the use of the medications. (Some medications may increase the breakdown rate of some neurotransmitters.)
- They don't restore balance to the excitatory/inhibitory systems.

Let's use the SSRIs as an example. After a neuron releases a neurotransmitter into a synapse, the chemical triggers a receptor site and then usually retreats back across the synapse, where it may be reabsorbed into the original neuron to be used again. If you take an SSRI, the drug blocks the reuptake (reabsorption) of the neurotransmitter, and the result is a temporary increase in the level of the chemical in the synapse. However, because it is in the synapse, it is subject to breakdown (metabolism). So long-term use of SSRIs can actually result in a lower level of neurotransmitters than you had before starting treatment.

That's not to say that psychotropic drugs should never be prescribed; if used judiciously, they can provide some benefit for some patients. However, the truth is that psychotropics often don't help patients for the reasons just stated. Therefore, *an orthomolecular approach is necessary if a healthy balance is to be achieved. Use of psychotropic drugs should be made on a patient-by-patient basis.*

## PSYCHOTROPICS AND AMINO ACID THERAPY

Although I do not routinely prescribe antidepressants and other psychotropic drugs as treatment for mood disorders, I do find that, when used judiciously in some patients, they are beneficial. One of the biggest arguments for the use of amino acid therapy instead of antidepressants and other psychotropic drugs is that the latter are not designed to increase neurotransmitter levels in the brain; amino acid therapy is. Thus, amino acid therapy seems the logical choice. However, the truth is many patients who come to me are already taking one or more psychotropics. Even though they tell me that the drugs are not working for them, I cannot simply tell them to stop taking them.

My goal when working with such individuals is to *gradually* wean them off their drugs once they have started amino acid therapy, along with other therapies as appropriate. I've found that use of a well-designed amino acid therapy program along with psychotropic drugs typically results in patients being able to reduce and ultimately eliminate their use of the drugs. This process is different for each patient: Some are able to cease use of their medications within a few short months, while others reduce their doses and continue their drugs while taking amino acids as well. Although there are exceptions to every rule, I generally do not begin tapering medications until I begin to see a favorable response to the nutrients over a four-week period.

Generally, nutrient therapy, including targeted amino acids, can be used very successfully in patients who are taking SSRIs, SNRIs (serotonin-norepinephrine reuptake inhibitors), antipsychotics, antiseizure medications, and antimanics (but not MAOIs), ultimately resulting in some individuals being able to stop their drug regimen altogether. Amino acid therapy can also increase the effectiveness of thyroid medications, especially those that require frequent dose adjustments. It also increases sensitivity to hormone replacement therapy, making it possible for individuals to reduce their reliance on such therapy.

If you go to a health-care practitioner who will test your neurotransmitter levels, it's important that you tell him or her all the medications you are taking, because some medications can influence neurotransmitter levels in the urine. It usually is not necessary to stop your medication to take part in neurotransmitter testing.

## ANTIDEPRESSANTS

We physicians have dozens of antidepressants we can prescribe for treatment of depression and other mood disorders. Some of these drugs have been available for decades, while others are relatively new to the market, yet typically they all share a promise of relieving symptoms of depression. The antidepressants designed to fulfill this promise fall into five main categories (see the table on pages 317 and 318 for a summary of brands and generics):

- Selective serotonin reuptake inhibitors (SSRIs).
- Mixed neurotransmitter reuptake inhibitors.
- Receptor blockers.
- Combination of reuptake inhibitor and receptor blocker.
- Enzyme inhibitors.

Any given type of antidepressant may perform one or more of the following actions:

- Block the activity of certain chemical receptors that neurotransmitters react with, which prevents nerve cells from receiving certain signals from other nerve cells.
- Inhibit the reuptake of one or more neurotransmitters, which keeps the neurotransmitters in the synapse for a longer time, and keeps them active until the supply is exhausted or new ones are produced.
- Inhibit monoamine oxidase enzymes that break down neurotransmitters, which means the neurotransmitters can remain in the synapse for a longer time.

## Antidepressants

|  | Generic | Trade Name(s) |
|---|---|---|
| **SSRIs** | Citalopram | Celexa |
|  | Fluoxetine | Prozac |
|  | Fluvoxamine | Luvox |
|  | Paroxetine | Paxil |
|  | Escitalopram | Lexapro |
|  | Sertraline | Zoloft |
| **Mixed reuptake inhibitors** | Bupropion | Wellbutrin |
|  | Venlafaxine | Effexor |
| **Receptor blockers** | Mirtazapine | Remeron |
| **Reuptake inhibitors and receptor blockers** | Amitriptyline | Elavil, Endep |
|  | Desipramine | Norpramin |
|  | Imipramine | Tofranil |

## **Antidepressants** (continued)

| | Generic | Trade Name(s) |
|---|---|---|
| | Maprotiline | Ludiomil |
| | Nefazodone | Serzone |
| | Nortriptyline | Aventyl, Pamelor |
| | Protriptyline | Vivactil |
| | Trazodone | Desyrel |
| | Trimipramine | Surmontil |
| **Monoamine oxidase enzyme inhibitors** | Phenelzine | Nardil |
| | Tranylcypromine | Parnate |

## Deadly Risks Associated with Antidepressant Use

That being said, I want to reiterate some critical information about antidepressants that was discussed in chapter 1: In some cases, their use has been associated with an increased risk of worsening symptoms of depression, suicide, and self-harm. The Food and Drug Administration has stated that "Patients with major depressive disorder (MDD), both adult and pediatric, may experience worsening of their depression and/or the emergence of suicidal ideation and behavior (suicidality) or unusual changes in behavior, whether or not they are taking antidepressant medications, and this risk may persist until significant remission occurs."

Generally, this has been the position of pharmaceutical companies, which have emphasized that it is the depressive illness itself that results in a worsening of symptoms, suicidality, and even homicidality, and not the drugs. However, much evidence indicates that this is not so—that in some patients, the medications themselves may increase the risks of these behaviors. The FDA finally acknowledged this possibility and, in April 2004, requested (but did not *require*) that manufacturers of antidepressants place a black box warning on their drugs, which is an alert to consumers that a drug carries a significant risk.

The FDA also recommended that doctors who are treating children with antidepressants monitor them closely for symptoms such as agitation, irritability, and unusual behavior changes, especially during the first few months of drug therapy or when dosages are changed. Ideally, monitoring should include face-to-face visits between the doctor and patient or the family weekly for the first four weeks, then one visit every other week for four weeks, then at least every twelve weeks, as long as the patient remains on the medication.

Such recommendations seem especially critical in light of information showing that some of the adolescents involved in school shootings in the past few years were taking Prozac. These included Kip Kinkel, who killed his parents and classmates in Oregon in 1998; Eric Harris, one of the shooters at Columbine in 1999; and Jeff Weise, the assailant in the Red Lake shootings in March 2005. Prior to the March 2005 incident, concerns about violence related to use of Prozac and other SSRIs prompted Health Canada (but not the FDA), in May 2004, to require warning labels on these drugs. The warning is: "There are clinical trial and post-marketing reports that SSRIs and other newer antidepressants, in both pediatrics and adults, of severe agitation-type adverse events coupled with self-harm or harm to others."

## Antidepressants and Withdrawal Symptoms

Another area of concern recently is the phenomenon of withdrawal symptoms that may occur when a patient tries to stop taking some of the newer antidepressants. Most psychiatrists have generally regarded the SSRIs as safer than some older types of antidepressants (the tricyclics and MAOIs), because they tend not to cause adverse cardiovascular side effects and death. In general, the newer antidepressants, when taken by themselves, don't cause death even with an overdose, while an overdose of older antidepressants often did cause death. Early promotional material on the newer antidepressants indicates that they are not addicting like the antianxiety benzodiazepines (such as Valium or Xanax).

However, we now know that the newer antidepressants can cause significant neurological and psychiatric symptoms such as anxiety and agitation when individuals try to go off them, especially if they stop suddenly. Everyone who takes antidepressants needs to be aware of this. Sometimes people try to stop one of these drugs and develop such severe symptoms that they return to the drug and are afraid to try stopping again. At times, psychiatrists will reinforce remaining on the medication, telling patients that the anxiety or agitation or neurological symptom responses prove they really need the medication and that these symptoms returned because they have stopped the drug. In my experience, these are *withdrawal* symptoms, as evidenced by the fact that when the patient slowly tapers the dosage while also trying to balance the neurotransmitters with targeted amino acids and other natural substances, the withdrawal symptoms can usually be minimized or eliminated. If you want to stop an antidepressant, you should do so under the guidance of a physician or psychiatrist who understands the withdrawal phenomenon and is able to support you nutritionally during the tapering process.

Clearly, antidepressant use should not be treated lightly. If you are already using antidepressants or your health-care provider wants to prescribe them, I suggest you talk to him or her about the natural alternatives discussed elsewhere in this book, as well as learning all you can about any antidepressant that may be included as part of your treatment plan. Here is a brief description of the different types of antidepressants.

## Selective Serotonin Reuptake Inhibitors

In the late 1980s, the first selective serotonin reuptake inhibitors (SSRIs) were introduced to the market. Scientists designed these drugs to work almost exclusively with serotonin and have little impact on other neurotransmitters. Current SSRIs include citalopram (Celexa), escitalopram (Lexapro), fluvoxamine (Luvox), fluoxetine (Prozac), paroxetine (Paxil), and sertraline (Zoloft).

Side effects associated with SSRIs include gastrointestinal problems, reduced libido and an inability to achieve an orgasm in both men and women (in about 30 percent of patients), anxiety, nervousness, headache, slight weight loss, rash, and insomnia.

### Drug Interactions

SSRIs cause a variety of reactions when they are taken with other medications. A partial list of those interactions is offered here. Consult with your doctor, pharmacist, and/or a reputable drug guide for more information on possible interactions.

• **Tricyclic and tetracyclic antidepressants.** Can cause

abnormal heart rhythms and an increase in tricyclic and tetra-cyclic levels.

• **SSRIs.** Increase in SSRI blood levels when more than one SSRI is taken.

• **MAOIs.** A rare but potentially deadly side effect is serotonin syndrome, characterized by confusion, hallucinations, fever, seizures, fluctuations in heart rhythm and blood pressure, and coma.

• **Serotonin antagonists**, such as trazodone (Desyrel) and nefazodone (Serzone). Increase in blood levels of trazodone and nefazodone, leading to anxiety.

• **Bupropion (Wellbutrin).** Increased risk of seizures.

• **Venlafaxine (Effexor).** May increase levels of venlafaxine.

• **Tolbutamine and insulin.** Causes low blood sugar.

• **Benzodiazepines**, including alprazolam (Xanax) and diazepam (Valium), among others. Confusion or excessive drowsiness, levels of benzodiazepines may increase.

• **Major tranquilizers** such as haloperidol (Haldol) and perphenazine (Trilafon). Blood levels of the tranquilizers may increase and cause increased side effects.

• **Warfarin (Coumadin).** Fluvoxamine may increase levels of warfarin and the risk of bleeding.

## Mixed Neurotransmitter Reuptake Inhibitors

Drugs in this category interfere with the reuptake of several neurotransmitters. Venlafaxine (Effexor) inhibits the reuptake of serotonin, dopamine, and norepinephrine. Use of this drug is associated with an increase in blood pressure. Along with depression, it is also used to treat obsessive-compulsive disorder.

Common side effects include anxiety, constipation, delayed orgasm, breathing difficulty, dizziness, dry mouth, itching, nausea, sedation, rash, sleep problems, vomiting, and unusual dreams.

Bupropion (Wellbutrin) inhibits the reuptake of dopamine and norepinephrine. It is used to treat major depression, attention deficit hyperactivity disorder (ADHD), and bipolar disorder. The most common side effects are insomnia (greater than 30 percent of users) and dry mouth; less common are dizziness, muscle pain, rash, itching, and change in appetite. Although it's less likely to cause the rise in blood pressure, sexual problems, drowsiness, or weight gain associated with SSRIs, it does increase the risk of seizures.

## Receptor Blockers

Thus far, the only FDA-approved receptor blocker for the treatment of depression is mirtazapine (Remeron), which prevents neurotransmitters from attaching themselves to nerve cell receptors that take signals from norepinephrine. This activity is believed to increase serotonin and norepinephrine activity in the brain. Mirtazapine appears to be especially helpful in depressed patients who have significant anxiety and/or insomnia.

Side effects of mirtazapine include sedation (occurs in more than 50 percent of users), weight gain, dry mouth, dizziness, light-headedness, thirst, joint and muscle aches, increased cholesterol, constipation, and increased appetite. Because it is less likely to cause sexual side effects, it is sometimes prescribed for patients who have had this problem with other antidepressants.

## Reuptake Inhibitors and Receptor Blockers

Antidepressants in this category perform two functions: They inhibit the reuptake of one or more neurotransmitters, and they block one or more nerve cell receptors. Included in this category are the following:

• **Tricyclic antidepressants**, which inhibit the reuptake of serotonin and norepinephrine and also block certain receptors. Each tricyclic functions in a slightly different way. Because they are associated with significant side effects (dry mouth, blurry vision, dizziness, drowsiness, constipation, difficulty urinating, weight gain, cardiac arrhythmias), they usually are not prescribed unless other antidepressants have not been effective, although low doses of some, such as Elavil, are sometimes prescribed before the newer ones. Tricyclics include amitriptyline (Elavil, Endep), desipramine (Norpramin), imipramine (Tofranil), nortriptyline (Aventyl, Pamelor), protriptyline (Vivactil), and trimipramine (Surmontil).

• **Maprotiline (Ludiomil)**, which inhibits the reuptake of norepinephrine and blocks certain norepinephrine receptors.

• **Nefazodone (Serzone)**, which inhibits the reuptake of serotonin and norepinephrine, and blocks a particular type of serotonin receptor and norepinephrine receptor.

• **Trazodone (Desyrel)**, which inhibits the reuptake of serotonin and blocks a type of serotonin receptor as well as several kinds of norepinephrine and histamine receptors. Because it blocks histamine receptors, it is more likely to cause drowsiness than other antidepressants, and so some physicians use it as a sleep aid.

## Monoamine Oxidase Enzyme Inhibitors

Antidepressants in this category are known as monoamine oxidase inhibitors, or MAOIs. These drugs, which include phenelzine (Nardil) and tranylcypromine (Parnate), block the action of monoamine oxidase enzymes, which break down serotonin and norepinephrine. The result is that these neurotransmitters remain active in the synapse longer. MAOIs are seldom prescribed today, however, because they can cause a rapid rise in blood pressure, which can lead to headache, rapid heartbeat, and possibly a stroke if they are used along with foods that contain the amino acid tyramine, which is present in cheese, chocolate, soy foods, avocados, coffee, beer, red wine, pickles, and other foods.

## OTHER PSYCHOTROPICS

Several other types of psychotropic drugs are frequently prescribed for symptoms of mood disorders, sometimes alone but often along with one or more antidepressants. These psychotropics work by interfering with the function of various neurotransmitter receptors, depending on the drug used.

### Antianxiety Drugs

Also known as sedatives or anxiolytics, drugs in this category include alprazolam (Xanax), buspirone (BuSpar), clonazepam (Klonopin), diazepam (Valium), and lorazepam (Ativan). Most of these drugs are benzodiazepines (except buspirone) and are characterized by rapid response: You can expect to experience results about thirty minutes after taking a dose. Because antidepressants can take several weeks to take effect, some doctors prescribe a benzodiazepine at the same time to help control anxiety until the antidepressant begins to control symptoms.

Benzodiazepines have several drawbacks, including a tendency to become habit forming. Side effects include dizziness, drowsiness, loss of balance, and reduced muscle coordination. Many other drug–drug interactions are possible, so please check with your health-care practitioner before using anti-anxiety drugs along with any other medications or supplements. Buspirone, which can take two to three weeks to take effect, can cause light-headedness, as well as headache, nausea, and nervousness.

## Mood Stabilizers

These drugs are typically taken to treat bipolar disorder, a condition characterized by episodes of mania and depression (see chapter 3). Mood-stabilizing drugs include lithium (Eskalith, Lithobid) and antiseizure drugs such as valproic acid (Depakote) and carbamazepine (Carbatrol, Tegretol). Lithium can cause nausea, excessive urination, diarrhea, confusion, fatigue, thyroid inhibition, and trembling hands. Psychiatrists sometimes prescribe antiseizure medications along with lithium for better control of mood swings. Side effects of valproic acid can include increased appetite, weight gain, digestive problems, and sedation, while carbamazepine can cause rash, dizziness, drowsiness, confusion, headache, and nausea.

Psychiatrists also prescribe two newer antiseizure drugs, gabapentin (Neurontin) and lamotrigine (Lamictal), to treat mood disorders, although as of this writing only Lamictal has been approved by the FDA to help prevent manic episodes, after standard treatment is used for the acute episode. Side effects of lamotrigine include dizziness, double vision, nausea, vomiting, and lack of muscle coordination. Serious skin conditions can occur, so the drug should be stopped at the first sign of a new rash. Side effects of gabapentin include sleepiness, dizziness, unsteadiness, fatigue, nausea, tremor, and double vision.

## Dilantin

For more than seventy years, physicians have used Dilantin (phenytoin) to treat epilepsy. Yet at least one person, notably Jack Dreyfus, founder of the Dreyfus Fund, experienced dramatic results with low doses of phenytoin for depression and obsessive negative thoughts. He was so impressed with this experience that he established a research foundation to study the effects of low-dose phenytoin on psychiatric conditions and wrote a book titled *The Story of a Remarkable Medicine.*

Another result was an indication that in relatively low doses (compared with doses used to control seizures), phenytoin helped to quiet excessive electrical activity in the brain. Such activity can be associated with rage reactions, impaired attention, anxiety, hyperactivity, bulimia, obsessive-compulsive symptoms, and others.

Dreyfus tried to stimulate interest in this alternative use of the medication among physicians, the drug manufacturer (Parke-Davis), the FDA, and politicians, but with little success. Parke-Davis was not interested in seeking new uses for the drug because the patent had run out and there was no financial incentive to do so. Julian Whitaker, MD, highlighted the use of low-dose phenytoin for psychiatric symptoms in his newsletter *Health & Healing*, reporting great success. Although I have not used low-dose phenytoin for psychiatric conditions, I would seriously consider it for patients presenting difficult cases whom I had not helped with other approaches.

## Stimulants

Drugs in this category include amphetamine (Adderall), dextroamphetamine (Dexedrine), and methylphenidate (Concerta, Metadate, Ritalin). Although they are used primarily as treatment for attention deficit hyperactivity disorder, they are also prescribed for some individuals who have not responded to other antidepressants. Stimulants have a chemical structure similar to that of dopamine and norepinephrine, and so they work by helping to increase the levels of these neurotransmitters in the brain. Use of stimulants along with other prescription and over-the-counter medication should be supervised by your doctor. Side effects of stimulant use include nervousness, sleep disturbances, headache, loss of appetite, stomach pain, abnormal heart rhythms, and weight loss.

If you have any of the following medical conditions or situations, you should talk to your health-care practitioner before taking a stimulant, as it may cause serious problems. Those conditions include current or past alcohol or drug abuse, severe anxiety or depression, seizure disorder, heart or blood vessel disease, high blood pressure, glaucoma, hyperthyroidism, or psychosis or other severe mental illness.

Stimulants may also interact negatively with many other medications, including but not limited to other stimulants, caffeine, diet pills, beta-blockers (such as Inderal, Lopressor, Tenormin), thyroid hormones, cold/allergy/asthma/sinus medications (prescription and over the counter), and tricyclic antidepressants.

## Antipsychotics

Antipsychotics are usually prescribed for depressed individuals who have severe depression and psychosis, a condition characterized by delusions or hallucinations. The most common antipsychotics include the old standby haloperidol (Haldol) and the newer atypical antipsychotics clozapine (Clozaril), olanzapine (Zyprexa), quetiapine (Seroquel), risperidone (Risperdal), and ziprasidone (Geodon). They work by blocking the effects of dopamine on certain dopamine receptors associated with psychosis. Among the side effects are weight gain, dry mouth, drowsiness, blurry vision, and constipation. Problems with glucose regulation leading to diabetes appears to be a serious long-term side effect of some if not all of these atypical antipsychotic medications. Users of antipsychotics also risk developing a rare but life-threatening condition called neuroleptic malignant syndrome, characterized by fever, rapid heartbeat, breathing difficulties, rigid muscles, irregular blood pressure, and convulsions. Also possible, especially among the elderly, is tardive dyskinesia, a condition in which people engage in lip smacking, involuntary movements, and worm-like movements of the tongue.

## THE BOTTOM LINE

Antidepressants and other psychotropic drugs have been a mainstay of treatment for depression and other mood disorders for decades, and—given the power of the pharmaceutical industry—it is unlikely they will disappear from the therapeutic scene in the near future. The emergence of amino acid therapy and evidence of its efficacy in the treatment of depression, however, is attracting the attention of physicians and the public, who are eager for a safe and effective treatment alternative. Therefore, we are fortunate that the vast majority of psychotropic medications work in harmony with amino acid therapy—a relationship that could make the transition to a natural approach to depression treatment an easier task.

## Chapter 13

*Chapter 13*

# Stories of Success

You've met many people throughout this book, and I've shared portions of their stories and how we treated their depressive symptoms. In this chapter, I present three more stories, but this time I include a more in-depth look at each individual's history, presenting complaints, test results, and treatment plan. Although each of these people has unique characteristics, they, like you and everyone else, possess the capacity to beat depression and to heal physically, emotionally, mentally, and spiritually. What an orthomolecular approach to depression does is tap into and nurture this capacity, as you'll see in the stories that follow.

## GERALDINE'S STORY

Geraldine, a fifty-six-year-old registered nurse and grandmother of three, first came to the Schachter Center in July 2004 after she was referred by her personal trainer. Her main complaints at the time, as she related them to our certified physician assistant Sally Minniefield, were periodic depression, panic attacks, and anxiety, along with menopausal symptoms that included night sweats, vaginal dryness, low sexual drive, and hot flashes. The depression, she said, "has been a persistent problem for about ten years. I get so depressed for at least a day or two every week, and I just have no desire to do anything. It's a struggle to get out of bed. I don't even feel like seeing my grandchildren when I'm that low." She also reported a long history of sleep difficulties, which included waking up every two to three hours and then finding it hard to go back to sleep. She felt that her poor sleep was "probably the reason why I'm always so tired. I've been tired for about ten years," she said, "and it affects my ability to concentrate."

In March 2002, Geraldine had been diagnosed with post-traumatic stress disorder after a close friend of hers was killed in an automobile accident, in a vehicle in which Geraldine was also a passenger. (Geraldine escaped with minor injuries.) Her general practitioner prescribed Prozac to help her cope with the anxiety and panic attacks she was experiencing, but Geraldine stopped taking it within twenty-four hours because she said it made her feel "spaced out." Both the anxiety and panic attacks gradually subsided on their own, but her depression persisted.

Geraldine told Ms. Minniefield that her diet had "always been rather good," and included organic foods whenever possible. This included one cup of organic coffee each morning and two glasses of organic white wine before going to bed, the latter a habit she had had for at least ten years. She also confessed to having a sweet tooth that she satisfied daily with chocolate "of any kind, from candy to ice cream to cookies."

Stating that she was "tired of feeling so low," in summer 2003 Geraldine decided to "take the bull by the horns" and instituted some changes to her life. After reading about the relationship between nutrition and mood, she added a long list of supplements to her program, including a multivitamin/mineral, calcium (700 mg) and magnesium (400 mg), a B-complex, ester C (1,000 mg), chromium (500 mcg), vitamin E (400 IU), coenzyme Q10 (100 mg), milk thistle (900 mg), chlorella (10 small tablets), flaxseed/fish oil (1 tablespoon), carotenoids, and whey protein. In winter 2004, she began working with a personal trainer one day a week, and then increased it to twice a week. She said she felt the supplements and exercise "had helped a bit," but "obviously not nearly enough, or else I wouldn't be here."

During the remainder of her first visit, Geraldine told Ms. Minniefield that she had had Epstein-Barr syndrome diagnosed in 1998, and it had taken her many months to recover. Since the onset of menopause she had used conventional hormone replacement therapy occasionally and it sometimes helped, but she decided to stop it in 2003 after research suggested it might be associated with an increased risk of breast cancer. She said she had never had any allergies, and, except for six mercury amalgam fillings, her physical examination did not reveal anything else of note.

Based on the information she collected during the initial visit, Ms. Minniefield suggested that Geraldine maintain her current supplement program but increase her vitamin E intake by 400 IU and begin taking evening primrose oil (1,300 mg) and theanine with GABA to help her sleep. She also recommended Geraldine follow my "Foods to Avoid" list (see chapter 7), which meant she should eliminate sweets and wine, among other items, and continue with her exercise program. Ms. Minniefield ordered laboratory tests and asked Geraldine to return in three weeks (mid-August 2004) to get the results and to consult with me.

Because of a family emergency, Geraldine was not able to return for her second visit until early November. At that time she met with me and explained that her priorities were to "lose the weight I've gained over the past year, get rid of this depression, and regain my sex drive." She also complained that she had been experiencing painful intercourse, which had been present for at least four years and was getting worse. Brief use of Prempro (a combination of horse-urine-based estrogen and a synthetic progestin) a few years before had made intercourse somewhat less painful but had done nothing for her sex drive, so she discontinued using it around the time the adverse effects of this drug were publicized.

Geraldine and I reviewed her laboratory test results. She had low estrone and progesterone, low epinephrine and serotonin, but elevated norepinephrine, dopamine, GABA, glutamate, and phenylethylamine (PEA), which suggested overactivity of the excitatory neurotransmitters. Since the first thing we wanted to do was balance her inhibitory neurotransmitters, I started her on a six-week program of an amino acid product that includes 5-HTP (to boost serotonin levels) and theanine, which has a calming effect and would help with her sleep difficulties. To help balance her hormones, I prescribed bioidentical progesterone cream (20 mg daily) and bioidentical oral estriol capsules (1.5 mg twice daily) from a compounding pharmacy, which she took on days one through twenty-five of each month. To improve her sex drive, I recommended a proprietary herbal preparation that contains chrysin, muira puama, and other herbs that inhibit the conversion of testosterone into estrogen, thus increasing dihydrotestosterone (DHT) levels. She was instructed to return in six weeks.

At her next visit six weeks later right before Christmas, Geraldine reported that her sleep "was so much better, and is still improving." She still experienced some night sweats, but they had improved as well. At that point, I adjusted Geraldine's treatment to include formulas designed to further support the inhibitory neurotransmitters, reduce GABA excretion, reduce norepinephrine and epinephrine activity, and support transsulfuration and methylation. The preparations contained taurine, theanine, glutamine, N-acetylcysteine (NAC), 5-HTP, vitamin $B_6$, folic acid, vitamin $B_{12}$, zinc, selenium, and other nutrients to support transsulfuration, methylation, and production of glutathione.

By late January 2005, Geraldine said her vaginal dryness was gone and painful intercourse had improved about 50 percent. She also reported having "great sleep, and this is such a gift," along with no more depressive episodes, much more energy, a sense of well-being and calm, and return of mental clarity.

A review and comparison of Geraldine's test results from July 2004 and January 2005 show a significant improvement in serotonin, dopamine, norepinephrine, glutamate, and PEA, as well as estrone, progesterone, and cortisol. In January 2005, her DHT was still low and her testosterone remained high. Although a few more minor adjustments needed to be made to her treatment plan, Geraldine had improved, by her own account, "about 200 percent" and could look forward to more improvement in the coming months as we continued to make adjustments to her treatment and monitor her with neurotransmitter tests every three months.

# Geraldine's Test Results

## Urine Neurotransmitter Test Results

|  | Optimal | 7/2004 | 1/2005 |
|---|---|---|---|
| Epinephrine | 8–12 | 5.2 | 5.3 |
| Norepinephrine | 30–55 | 83 | 57 |
| Dopamine | 125–175 | 204.6 | 131.9 |
| Serotonin | 175–225 | 108.9 | 325.1 |
| GABA | 2–4 | 5.5 | 5.9 |
| Glutamate | 10–25 | 43.2 | 36.6 |
| PEA | 175–350 | 480–487 | 310.6 |
| Histamine | 10–22 | 12.5 | 25.1 |

## Saliva Hormone Test Results

| | | | |
|---|---|---|---|
| Estradiol | 1–2 | 1.2 | 1.4 |
| Estrone | 1–3 | 0.8 | 1.4 |
| Progesterone | 0.2–0.5 | 0.05 | 1.9 |
| Testosterone | 15–35 | 45.7 | 54.3 |
| Dihydrotestosterone (DHT) | 5–12 | 4.5 | 3.8 |
| DHEA | 300–500 | 410.6 | 384.2 |
| Cortisol 7 AM | 8–15 | 6.1 | 11 |
| Cortisol 11 AM | 3–7 | 1.4 | 3.9 |
| Cortisol 3 PM | 2–4 | 7.2 | 2.2 |
| Cortisol 7 PM | 0.3–1.5 | 0.7 | 0.6 |

## MURRAY'S STORY

When Murray first came to the Schachter Center in October 2004, his story was like that of many other patients: He was being treated for several different medical and psychiatric problems with various drugs. Whenever patients are taking many different medications, the combinations can contribute to other problems. Such was the case with Murray.

At age forty-six, Murray was married with two teenage sons, significantly overweight, and out of work on disability leave because of depression and a chronic pain condition in his knee. For more than a year, he had tried various treatments for the pain, including acupuncture, glucosamine with chondroitin, morphine, and fentanyl (an opioid for severe pain), but he had experienced little or no relief through any of these options, and severe constipation through use of morphine. When he walked into my center, he was considering a recent suggestion by his orthopedic specialist to undergo knee surgery.

The history he gave to our certified physician's assistant John Reynolds was, in Murray's words, "pretty depressing." At age thirty-seven, Murray had had a heart attack in which his right coronary artery had been nearly 100 percent blocked. The artery was cleared with balloon angioplasty, but within a year he had to return to the hospital because of heart pain (angina), and two other coronary arteries were found to be nearly completely blocked. These were treated with stents (flexible tubes), and Murray was sent home with multiple heart medications, including simvastatin to reduce his cholesterol level, isosorbide to dilate his coronary arteries, and a baby aspirin to help prevent blood clots. He was also taking metoprolol and lisinopril for his high blood pressure. Fortunately, this treatment plan had continued to work for Murray for more than eight years, and he had not experienced any heart problems since receiving the stents.

Therefore, his main complaints when he came to the Schachter Center were long-standing depression and knee pain. In fact, Murray had been diagnosed with depression back when he was nineteen and had been on the antidepressant paroxetine from ages thirty-two to forty-four, when, he said, "I decided I had had enough of drugs. I needed to take the heart and blood pressure medications, so the only thing I thought I could stop was the antidepressant." Beginning in March 2003, he slowly reduced the dosage, until by midsummer he was completely off the drug. "It wasn't easy," he said. "I experienced a lot of light-headedness and a whooshing sound when I turned my head. Sometimes I heard sounds. But I got through it."

Murray said he felt fine for about a month after ending the paroxetine, but then he became severely depressed and anxious, and he was hospitalized on a psychiatric inpatient unit in the fall for two months. During that time he was given bupropion and then paroxetine again, but he did not respond. (His lack of response to these drugs was likely due to an extremely low serotonin level—even though it had not been measured at the time—which was likely the result of his long-term use of paroxetine.) His psychiatrist recommended electroconvulsive therapy (ECT), which involves attaching electrodes to an individual's head while he or she is under anesthesia. An electric shock is administered to the head, which causes the patient to experience a seizure for less than a minute. This treatment is frequently recommended when a patient with severe depression does not respond to drug treatment. The main side effect of ECT is memory impairment, which is usually temporary but can persist indefinitely in some individuals. Murray underwent six ECT sessions over a two-week period while in the hospital, after which his depression had improved enough for him to be released home. He received another twelve ECT sessions as an outpatient over the next several months, for eighteen treatments in all.

Once Murray completed the ECT sessions, he began to see another psychiatrist, who continued Murray on the bupropion and paroxetine but added lithium carbonate to stabilize his mood, and clonazepam, an antianxiety drug. The lithium caused Murray to experience tremors and cluster headaches, and he stopped taking it. After trying this drug combination for several months and not noticing any significant improvement, Murray sought help at our center in October 2004.

One very positive note that was revealed during Murray's initial visit was that he had recently started exercising several times a week: thirty minutes on a stationary bicycle three times a week and fifteen minutes of swimming twice a week. He also was lifting weights and was able to press significant weight with his legs.

Once John Reynolds collected Murray's extensive history during the first visit, he ordered a series of tests, including a urine neurotransmitter test and serum testosterone levels—he suspected that Murray had low levels of this hormone given his hot flashes and fatigue. When the results came back, we found that Murray indeed had severe imbalances in neurotransmitter levels (see the table on page 342) and a very low serum testosterone level of 300 (400 to 700 is normal). We immediately started him on two amino acid formulas designed to enhance the inhibitory neurotransmitter system (improve serotonin and GABA functioning). They contain 5-HTP, vitamins and minerals that stimulate conversion to serotonin, taurine, theanine, and other amino acids. To help correct the low testosterone level, Murray was given a transdermal testosterone cream to apply daily.

When Murray arrived for his next visit in late November 2004, six weeks after he had started treatment, he was a different man. "I haven't felt this good in years," he said. "I felt remarkably better within five days of starting the amino acids and the testosterone. I can't believe it." At this point, we initiated the second phase of treatment, in which we enhance the excitatory neurotransmitters. This involved stopping one of the first two amino acid formulas and adding one that contained *Mucuna pruriens* to build dopamine, and *Rhodiola rosea* and histidine to enhance histamine production. He was also given NAC to improve methylation.

Within days, Murray was reporting even more improvement. "My fatigue is completely gone, and my depression is much better," he said. "And the testosterone has done wonders for my sex drive." Although he was still experiencing pain in his knee, Murray's mood was so improved he returned to work after being on disability for more than a year. When he went to his psychiatrist and told him about the neurotransmitter test and the amino acid therapy, the doctor was visibly upset and told Murray it was "all nonsense."

But Murray was not to be deterred. His next goal was to wean himself off his drugs, starting with bupropion. When I saw Murray at the end of January 2005, he had successfully withdrawn from bupropion and paroxetine and had reduced his simvastatin by half. He was still following the second phase of treatment he had started in late November 2004, and to this we added DHEA, a multivitamin/mineral, coenzyme Q10 (100 mg), SAMe (800 mg, to address abnormal liver enzymes— likely the result of irritation from all the medications Murray had been taking for so many years), fish oil, calcium, and magnesium. He said he was experiencing some sleeping problems, so we recommended 500 mg of L-tryptophan at bedtime and 1 to 3 tablespoons of flaxseed oil daily. We also ordered a retest of his neurotransmitter levels (see the 2/2005 results in the table on pages 341 and 342).

Murray had another visit in March 2005 and said his depression was much better. He had increased his CoQ10 to 300 mg daily, which seemed to result in improved kidney function. Since starting SAMe, his liver enzymes had improved. Murray's only complaints during this visit were that he was still having trouble falling asleep, and he was anxious in the morning. He came to see me in April and said that for the first time in seventeen years, he was not taking any antidepressants. He was still taking clonazepam or alprazolam for anxiety, however, and I noted that the anxiety he was experiencing in the morning could be related to withdrawal symptoms; a new goal would be to stop taking these medications as well. He agreed and said that his psychiatrist was still skeptical about what his patient was doing, even though it obviously was working.

The table on pages 341 and 342 gives you an indication of how well Murray was doing at his second neurotransmitter test in February 2005 as compared with his initial (baseline) test results. On the second test, all neurotransmitter levels were either optimal or greatly improved from baseline, with the most significant improvement being in serotonin.

(It is very possible that Murray's extremely low serotonin level at baseline was due to long-term use of antidepressants.) The fact that epinephrine had not improved more suggested there was a problem with methylation, and the less-than-optimal levels of norepinephrine and dopamine indicated Murray needed more support of the excitatory neurotransmitters. The fact that Murray was experiencing anxiety in the morning was not surprising given that his 7 AM cortisol level was high, and the dramatic drop in cortisol levels for the rest of the day suggested he needed adrenal support. His positive response to testosterone treatment and high saliva testosterone led us to reduce his dosage by 50 percent. (When testosterone is administered as a transdermal cream, however, saliva levels may overestimate tissue levels, while serum testosterone levels tend to underestimate them.)

## Murray's Test Results

### Urine Neurotransmitter Test Results

|  | Optimal | 10/2004 | 2/2005 |
|---|---|---|---|
| Epinephrine | 8–12 | 2.5 | 5.6 |
| Norepinephrine | 30–55 | 11.9 | 23.9 |
| Dopamine | 125–175 | 44 | 67.2 |
| Serotonin | 175–225 | 27.4 | 213.3 |
| GABA | 2–4 | 2.7 | 4.4 |
| Glutamate | 10–25 | 16.8 | 19.6 |
| PEA | 175–350 | 201.5 | 261.6 |
| Histamine | 10–22 | 17 | 18.6 |

## Murray's Test Results (continued)

### Saliva Hormone Test Results

|  | Optimal | 10/2004 | 2/2005 |
|---|---|---|---|
| DHEA (male) | 300–600 |  | 549.7 |
| Cortisol 7 AM | 8–15 |  | 21.9 |
| Cortisol noon | 3–7 |  | 0.8 |
| Cortisol 5 PM | 2–4 |  | 0.7 |
| Cortisol 10 PM | 0.3–1.5 |  | 0.3 |
| Estradiol | 0.8–1.5 |  | 0.4 |
| Estrone | 1–2.5 |  | 1.5 |
| Progesterone | 0.07–0.15 |  | 0.1 |
| Testosterone | 75–95 |  | 1,074.6 |
| DHT | 20–40 |  | 28.4 |

At Murray's April 2005 visit I added theanine spray to his program to alleviate his anxiety and to help him get off clonazepam. I also began to taper simvastatin (while monitoring his lipid levels), because he had complained of poor memory since his ECT sessions had stopped, and there is some evidence that statin drugs impair memory. Other plans for Murray consisted of repeating the urinary neurotransmitter and saliva tests about every three months several more times so we could make any additional adjustments in treatment. It was clear at the time of Murray's April 2005 visit that he had experienced a dramatic turnaround over the past six months and was still making significant improvements.

## LILA'S STORY

Lila is a forty-one-year-old single general practitioner who has a very successful group practice with three other physicians. She first came to the Schachter Center in March 2005 complaining of severe depression and anxiety and suicidal thoughts. She told our certified physician's assistant John Reynolds that she had experienced these feelings in the past, but that they had been very bad for the last six months. Recently, she was feeling overwhelmed by everything in her life, including her work, and she dreaded everything she had to do. She was able to identify the trigger for the latest severe bout of depression—a crisis in a ten-year relationship with her partner that culminated in her partner leaving her in September 2004. Lila now lived alone in the apartment they had shared for a decade. Soon after the breakup Lila tried to cut herself, making a superficial slash on her wrist.

Prior to the current severe bout of depression, Lila said she had had a "nervous breakdown" in May 2004 at which time she had heard voices calling her "stupid" and other derogatory names. She went to see a psychiatrist, who prescribed the antipsychotic drug Zyprexa, but it caused her to feel too sleepy so she discontinued it. The voices eventually stopped on their own, but her depression got worse, especially after her partner left her. At that time, Lila began to see another psychiatrist once a month. This one prescribed Effexor (225 mg daily), lithium (900 mg daily, to improve the results of the Effexor), and Ativan (1 mg once or twice daily) for anxiety. She said, "I think the Ativan might be helping with the anxiety, but I don't think the other two are beneficial at all." She also began seeing a psychiatric social worker for psychotherapy once a week. At the time she came to the Schachter Center, she was still seeing both of these professionals.

When the physician's assistant asked Lila about her diet, she said she had lost about 25 pounds since her partner left. Her eating habits were highly erratic; she often skipped breakfast, ate a sandwich for lunch, and sometimes skipped dinner. "I just don't have much of an appetite," she said.

Concerning her emotional state, she said that she sometimes thinks about cutting herself, but she hasn't done it again. She has been able to continue working, and lately she was taking time to do an hour of yoga three or four times a week.

A physical examination was normal except for a slightly low blood pressure, dry skin, and several mercury amalgam fillings in her mouth. Mr. Reynolds ordered laboratory tests, including urine neurotransmitter and saliva hormone tests, and advised Lila to increase her calorie and protein intake and to follow the "Foods to Avoid" list (see chapter 7). He also started her on a complete high-quality multivitamin and -mineral supplement, along with fish oil capsules, and made an appointment for her to return in six weeks.

Two days after her first visit to the center, Mr. Reynolds called Lila and told her that her homocysteine level was very high (greater than 16, with normal being below 9) and that she should double her intake of the multivitamin and -mineral, which significantly increased her intake of folic acid and vitamins $B_6$ and $B_{12}$. This she did, and when she came for her next visit six weeks later in early May 2005, she said, "I began to feel better after being on the supplements for about three weeks, well enough to stop the Ativan. But the fish oil bothered my stomach, so I stopped taking it." Lila said she was eating much better than she had been; she was not skipping meals and was including protein and fruits and vegetables in her diet. She also expressed concern about taking the Effexor and lithium, both of which she wanted to stop. However, she said, "I'm too frightened to consider doing that just yet." I told her she would know when she was ready to gradually withdraw from these drugs.

Lila and I reviewed her laboratory results at that second visit, and they revealed why she was feeling so bad. Her serum vitamin $B_{12}$ level was very low (182, with normal being at least 300 to 400); her folic acid was borderline low at 8.6. Neither of which was surprising given that her homocysteine was very high. Her vitamin D level was extremely low at 7.8 (25-hydroxyvitamin D should be at least 30). Her blood count, comprehensive metabolic profile (which tests for liver and kidney function), and cholesterol were normal. Results of her red blood cell minerals showed elevated arsenic and low potassium and molybdenum.

Lila's urinary neurotransmitter results showed low epinephrine (indicating problems with methylation, also evident with her low $B_{12}$ and folic acid levels), low dopamine, very high histamine, and very low serotonin, which helps explain why the venlafaxine (Effexor) had not been helpful. My suggestions to her at this visit were as follows:

- Increase her sunlight exposure (without the use of sunscreen, but also without getting sunburned) to improve her very low vitamin D level, plus take 5,000 IU vitamin D daily for one month, then 2,000 IU daily.
- Get an injection of $B_{12}$ (1,000 mcg) at this visit and a subsequent one.

- Add more $B_6$, $B_{12}$, folic acid, and trimethylglycine to her supplement program to bring down her homocysteine level, improve methylation, and improve transsulfuration.
- Add flaxseed oil (1 to 2 tablespoons daily) to supply omega-3 fatty acids.
- Begin amino acid therapy to correct the inhibitory neurotransmitter deficiencies, to include 5-HTP, theanine, taurine, and acetylcysteine.

We will continue to monitor Lila's progress and make adjustments to her amino acid therapy and nutritional supplementation as needed. She and I are confident she will eventually stop both the lithium and venlafaxine. At future sessions, we will likely discuss her interest in possibly removing her mercury amalgam fillings.

# Closing Remarks

———————— ❧ ————————

We have now completed our journey into comprehensive and what I believe are exciting cutting-edge approaches in the evaluation and treatment of depression and other mood disorders. I have shared with you the methods I find most effective and safe in eliminating depression, methods that focus on an orthomolecular, self-healing philosophy. I have also tried to emphasize that many factors may contribute to depression and that a detailed and conscientious approach can be most helpful in ascertaining which of these factors are most important and relevant to treat in a particular individual. To that end, I have provided many tools you can use to help you beat depression and restore balance to your life.

Sometimes the elements and conditions that contribute to and cause depression are relatively simple to identify and correct, and individuals can successfully treat their own depressive symptoms by following some of the guidelines in this book. I sincerely hope you can count yourself in this group. At other times, professional help, sophisticated testing, and even medication may be necessary. In fact, if you have any doubts or questions about handling your own evaluation and treatment, I believe it is always better to err on the side of caution and seek professional guidance. If this is true for you, then I hope you will share the concepts in this book with your chosen health-care professionals and work together to dispel your depression. You should now have a much broader view of how depression can be evaluated and treated and of the types of diagnostic and therapeutic options available to you. The resources at the back of this book should be helpful as you determine the path you will take.

Every journey, no matter how long or short, easy or difficult, begins the same way: with one step. Congratulations: You've already taken that step by reading this book. Just keep walking.

# Selected Chapter Notes

---- ⚘ ----

## Introduction

Hoffer A. *Vitamin B-3 and Schizophrenia: Discovery, Recovery, Controversy.* Kingston, Ontario: Quarry Press, 1999.

*Journal of the American Medical Association* 2003 Jun 18. The entire issue is dedicated to depression.

## CHAPTER 1: What's Wrong with the Mainstream Approach to Treating Depression

Alliance for Human Research Protection, www.ahrp.org/informail/04/06/02.html.

AlternativeMedicine.com. *CFS, Fibromyalgia, and Lyme Disease.*

Brown RJ et al. Neurodynamics of relapse prevention: A neuro-nutrient approach to outpatient DUI offenders. *J Psychoactive Drugs* 1990 Apr–Jun; 22(2).

Burrascano JH. Lyme disease. In *Conn's Current Therapy*, RE Rakel, ed. Philadelphia: WB Saunders, 1997.

Caspi A et al. Influence of life stress on depression: Moderation by a polymorphism in the 5-HTT gene. *Science* 2003 Jul 18; 301(5631): 386–9.

Holick M. *The UV Advantage.* New York: I Books, Simon & Schuster, 2004.

IMS. US physicians responsive to patient requests for brand-name drugs. IMG press release, Apr 1, 2002, www.imshealth

.com/ims/portal/front/articleC/0,2777,6599_3665_1003811,00
.html.

Kramlinger K, ed. *Mayo Clinic on Depression*. Philadelphia: Mason Crest Publishers, 2001.

Lesperance F, Frasure-Smith N, Talajic M. Major depression before and after myocardial infarction: Its nature and consequences. *Psychosom Med* 1996; 58(2): 99–110.

Nemeroff CB, Musselman DL, Evans DL. Depression and cardiac disease. *Depression and Anxiety* 1998; 8(suppl 1): 71–9.

Nolen-Hoeksema S. The role of rumination in depressive disorders and mixed anxiety/depressive symptoms. *J Abnorm Psychol* 2000 Aug; 109(3): 504–11.

Philpott WH, Kalita DK, Pauling L. *Brain Allergies*. New York: McGraw-Hill, 2000.

Sanacora G et al. Subtype-specific alterations of gamma-amino-butyric acid and glutamate in patients with major depression. *Arch Gen Psychiatry* 2004; 61: 705–13.

Ward A et al. Can't quite commit: Rumination and uncertainty. *Pers Soc Psychol Bull* 2003 Jan; 29(1): 96–107.

Wassertheil-Smoller S et al. Depression and cardiovascular sequelae in postmenopausal women: The Women's Health Initiative (WHI). *Arch Intern Med* 2004 Feb 9; 164(3): 289–98.

Zito JM et al. Psychotropic practice patterns for youth and adolescents: A 10-year perspective. *Arch Ped Adolesc Med* 2003 Jan; 157(1): 17–25.

Zubenko GS et al. Genetic linkage of region containing the CREB1 gene to depressed disorders in women from families with recurrent, early-onset major depression. *Am J Med Genet* 2002 Dec 8; 114(8): 980–7.

———. Sequence variations in CREB1 cosegregate with depressive disorders in women. *Mol Psychiatry* 2003 Jun; 8(6): 611–8.

## CHAPTER 2: Why Are You Depressed?
## You Are What You Eat

Centers for Disease Control and Prevention, www.cdc.gov/od/oc/media/pressrel/r040121.htm.

Chemiske S. *Caffeine Blues: Wake Up to the Hidden Dangers of America's #1 Drug.* New York: Warner, 1998.

Christensen L. The roles of caffeine and sugar in depression. *Nutrition Report* 1991; 9(3): 17, 24.

Cousens G. *Depression-Free for Life.* New York: HarperCollins, 2000.

Food and Drug Administration, www.fda.gov/cder/news/phen/fenphenqa2.htm.

Ross J. *The Diet Cure.* New York: Penguin Putnam, 2000.

*Super Size Me* (DVD video). Sundance Video, Hart Sharp Video, 2004.


## CHAPTER 3: Discover Your Biochemical Profile and
## Get the Professional Help You Need

Cousens G. *Depression-Free for Life.* New York: HarperCollins, 2000.

Pfeiderer B et al. Effective electroconvulsive therapy reverse glutamate/glutamine deficit in the left anterior cingulum of unipolar depressed patients. *Psychiatry Res* 2003 Apr 1; 122(3): 185–92.

Shafii M et al. Nocturnal serum melatonin profile in major depression in children and adolescents. *Arch Gen Psychiatry* 1996; 53(11): 1009–13.

Thompson C et al. Effects of morning phototherapy on circadian markers in seasonal affective disorder. *Br J Psychiatry* 1997; 170: 431–5.


## CHAPTER 4: Up with Amino Acids

Argyropoulos SV et al. Tryptophan depletion reverses the therapeutic effect of SSRIs in social anxiety disorder. *Biol Psychiatry* 2004 Oct 1; 56(7): 503–9.

Baumel S. *Dealing with Depression Naturally.* New York: McGraw-Hill, 1995.

Birdsall TC. 5-hydroxytryptophan: A clinically-effective serotonin precursor. *Altern Med Rev* 1998 Aug; 3(4): 271–80.

Chadwick D, Jenner P, Harris R, et al. Manipulation of brain serotonin in the treatment of myoclonus. *Lancet* 1975; 2: 434–5.

Chaitow L. *Thorson's Guide to Amino Acids.* London: HarperCollins Publishing, 1991.

Chouinard G et al. A controlled clinical trial of L-tryptophan in acute mania. *Biol Psychiatry* 1985 May; 20: 546–57.

Den Boer JA, Westenberg HG. Behavioral, neuroendocrine, and biochemical effects of 5-hydroxytryptophan administration in panic disorder. *Psychiatry Res* 1990; 31: 267–78.

Kimura R, Murata T. Effect of theanine on norepinephrine and serotonin levels in rat brain. *Chem Pharm Bull (Tokyo)* 1986; 34(7): 3053–7.

Kobayashi K et al. Effects of L-theanine on the release of α-brain waves in human volunteers. *Nippon Nogeikagaku Kaishi* 1998; 72: 153–7.

Maar TE et al. Effects of taurine depletion on cell migration and NCAM expression in cultures of dissociated mouse cerebellum and N2A cells. *Amino Acids* 1998; 15(1–2): 77–88.

Maes M et al. Stimulatory effects of L-5-hydroxytryptophan on postdexamethasone beta-endorphin levels in major depression. *Neuropsychopharm* 1996; 15: 340–8.

Pöldinger W, Calanchini B, Schwarz W. A functional-dimensional approach to depression: Serotonin deficiency as a target syndrome in a comparison of 5-hydroxytryptophan and fluvoxamine. *Psychopathol* 1991; 24: 53–81.

Ross J. *The Mood Cure.* New York: Penguin, 2002.

Shealy C et al. The neurochemistry of depression. *Am J Pain Management* 2(1): 13–6.

Van Praag HM, Lemus C. Monoamine precursors in the treatment of psychiatric disorders. In *Nutrition and the Brain,* RJ Wurtman, JJ Wurtman, ed. New York: Raven Press, 1986: 89–139.

Yokogoshi H et al. Effect of theanine, γ-glutamylethylamide, on brain monoamines and striatal dopamine release in conscious rats. *Neurochem Res* 1998; 23(5): 667–73.

Yokogoshi H, Mochizuki M, Saitoh K. Theanine-induced reduction of brain serotonin concentration in rats. *Biosci Biotechnol Biochem* 1998; 62(4): 816–7.

## CHAPTER 5: Make the Most of Essential Fatty Acids and Other Fats

Adams PB, Lawson S, Sanigorski A, Sinclair AJ. Arachidonic acid to eicosapentaenoic acid ratio in blood correlates positively with clinical symptoms of depression. *Lipids* 1996 Mar; 31: S157–S161.

Balch JF, Stengler M. *Prescription for Natural Cures.* Hoboken, NJ: John Wiley & Sons, 2004.

Brambilla F, Maggioni M. Blood levels of cytokines in elderly patients with major depressive disorder. *Acta Psychiatr Scand* 1998; 97: 309–13.

Burdge GC et al. Eicosapentaenoic and docosapentaenoic acids are the principal products of alpha-linolenic acid metabolism in young men. *Br J Nutr* 2002; 88(4): 355–64.

Burdge GC, Wootton SA. Conversion of alpha-linolenic acid to eicosapentaenoic, docosapentaenoic and docosahexaenoic acids in young women. *Br J Nutr* 2002 88(4): 411–20.

Connor W. *Nutrition Action Health Letter* 2002 Jul–Aug: 6.

Ellis EF et al. Effect of dietary n-3 fatty acids on cerebra microcirculation. *Am J Physiol* 1992; 262: H1379–H1386.

Frasure-Smith N et al. Major depression is associated with lower omega-3 fatty acid levels in patients with recent acute coronary syndrome. *Biol Psychiatry* 2004 May 1; 55(9): 891–6.

Hibbeln JR. Chart of fish consumption and major depression. *Lancet* 1998.

———. Seafood consumption, the DHA content of mother's milk, and prevalence rates of postpartum depression. *J Affect Disord* 2002 May; 69(1–3): 15–29.

Ito H et al. Hypoperfusion in the limbic system and prefrontal cortex in depression: SPECT with anatomic standardization technique. *J Nucl Med* 1996; 37: 410–4.

Kimbrell TA et al. Regional cerebral glucose utilization in patients with a range of severities in unipolar depression. *Biol Psychiatry* 2002; 51: 237–52.

Logan AC. Neurobehavioral aspects of omega-3 fatty acids: Possible mechanisms and therapeutic value in major depression. *Altern Med Rev* 2003; 8: 410–25.

Maes M et al. Lowered n-3 polyunsaturated fatty acids in the serum phospholipids and cholesterol esters of depressed patients. *Psychiatry Res* 1999; 85: 275–91.

Maggioni M et al. Effects of phosphatidylserine therapy in geriatric patients with depressive disorders. *Acta Psychiatr Scand* 1990; 81: 265–70.

Mamalakis G, Tornaritis M, Kafatos A. Depression and adipose essential polyunsaturated fatty acids. *Prostaglandins Leukot Essent Fatty Acids* 2002; 67: 311–8.

Nemets B, Stahl Z, Belmaker RH. Addition of omega-3 fatty acid to maintenance medication treatment for recurrent unipolar depressive disorder. *Am J Psychiatry* 2002; 159: 477–9.

*Nutrition Science News*, July 2004, www.chiro.org/nutrition/FULL/Marine_vs_Veggie_Omega-3.html.

Peet M, Horrobin DF. A dose-ranging study of the effects of ethyl-eicosapentaenoate in patients with ongoing depression despite adequate treatment with standard drugs. *Arch Gen Psychiatry* 2002; 59: 913–9.

Peet M, Murphy B, Shay J, Horrobin D. Depletion of omega-3 fatty acid levels in red blood cell membranes of depressive patients. *Biol Psychiatry* 1998; 43: 315–9.

Sampalis F et al. Evaluation of the effects of Neptune krill oil on the management of premenstrual syndrome and dysmenorrhea. *Altern Med Rev* 2003;8(2): 171–9.

Severus WE, Ahrens B, Stoll A. Omega-3 fatty acids—the missing link? [letter]. *Arch Gen Psychiatry* 1999; 56: 380–1.

Simopoulos AP, Leaf A, Salem N. Workshop on the essentiality of and recommended dietary intakes for omega-6 and omega-3 fatty acids. *J Am Coll Nutr* 1999; 18: 487–9.

Stoll AL et al. Omega-3 fatty acids in bipolar disorder: A preliminary double-blind, placebo-controlled trial. *Arch Gen Psychiatry* 1999; 56: 407–12.

Su KP, Huang SY, Chiu CC, Shen WW. Omega-3 fatty acids in major depressive disorder: A preliminary double-blind, placebo controlled trial. *Eur Neuropsychopharmacol* 2003; 13: 267–71.

Tiemeier H et al. Plasma fatty acid composition and depression are associated in the elderly: The Rotterdam study. *Am J Clin Nutr* 2003; 78: 40–6.

De Wilde MC et al. The effect of n-3 polyunsaturated fatty acid-rich diets on cognitive and cerebrovascular parameters in chronic cerebral hypoperfusion. *Brain Res* 2002; 947: 166–73.

Zanarini MC, Frankenburg FR. Omega-3 fatty acid treatment of women with borderline personality disorder: A double-blind, placebo-controlled pilot study. *Am J Psychiatry* 2003; 160: 167–9.

Zimmer L et al. The dopamine mesocorticolimbic pathway is affected by deficiency in n-3 polyunsaturated fatty acids. *Am J Clin Nutr* 2002; 75: 662–7.

## CHAPTER 6: Lift Your Spirits with Nutrients and Herbs

Abraham GE. Iodine supplementation markedly increases urinary excretion of fluoride and bromide. *Townsend Letter* 2003; 238: 108–9.

————. The Wolff-Chaikoff effect of increasing iodide intake on the thyroid. *Townsend Letter* 2003; 245: 100–1.

————. The safe and effective implementation of orthoiodosupplementation in medical practice. *Original Internist* 2004; 11: 17–36.

Abraham GE, Flechas JD, Hakala JC. Orthoiodosupplementation: Iodine sufficiency of the whole human body. *Original Internist* 2002; 9: 30–41.

Arasteh K. A beneficial effect of calcium intake on mood. *J Orthomol Med* 1994: www.orthomed.org/links/papers/arastdep .htm.

Benton D, Cook R. The impact of selenium supplementation on mood. *Biol Psychiatry* 1991 Jun 1; 29(11): 1092–8.

Birkmayer W, Birkmayer JG. The coenzyme nicotinamide adenine dinucleotide (NADH) as biological antidepressive agent. *New Trends Clin Neuropharmacol* 1992; 5: 19–25.

Bradford GS, Taylor CT. Omeprazole and vitamin $B_{12}$ deficiency. *Ann Pharmacother* 1999 May; 33(5): 641–3.

Brink CB et al. Effects of myo-inositol versus fluoxetine and imipramine pretreatments on serotonin 5HT2A and muscarinic acetylcholine receptors in human neuroblastoma cells. *Metabol Brain Dis* 2004 Jun; 12(1–2): 51–70.

Brownstein D. *Iodine: Why You Need It, Why You Can't Live Without It.* West Bloomfield, MI: Medical Alternative Press, 2004.

Coppen A, Bailey J. Enhancement of the antidepressant action of fluoxetine by folic acid: A randomized placebo controlled trial. *J Affect Disord* 2000 Nov; 60(2): 121–30.

Davidson JR et al. Effectiveness of chromium in atypical depression: A placebo controlled trial. *Biol Psychiatry* 2003 Feb 1; 53(3): 261–4.

Einat H et al. Inositol reduces depressive-like behaviors in two different animal models of depression. *Psychopharmacology (Berl)* 1999 May; 144(2): 158–62.

Facchinetti F et al. Oral magnesium successfully relieves premenstrual mood changes. *Obstet Gynecol* 1991 Aug; 72(2): 177–81.

Holick M. *The UV Advantage.* New York: I Books, Simon & Schuster, 2004.

Hvas A-M et al. Vitamin $B_6$ level is associated with symptoms of depression. *Psychother Psychosom* 2005; 73: 340–3.

Hypericum Depression Trial Study Group. Effect of *Hypericum perforatum* (St. John's wort) in major depressive disorder: A randomized, controlled trial. *JAMA* 2002; 287: 1807–14.

Kelly GS. *Rhodiola rosea:* A possible plant adaptogen. *Altern Med Rev* 2001 Jun; 6(3): 293–302.

Kirby D. *Evidence of Harm: Mercury in Vaccines and the Autism Epidemic: A Medical Controversy.* New York: St. Martin's Press, 2005.

Levine J. Followup and relapse analysis of an inositol study of depression. *Israel J Psychiatry Rel Sci* 1995; 32: 14–21.

———. Controlled trials of inositol in psychiatry. *Eur Neuropsychopharmacol* 1997; 7(2): 147–55.

Linde K et al. St. John's wort for depression: An overview and meta-analysis of randomised clinical trials. *BMJ* 1996 Aug 3; 313(7052): 253–8.

Loma Linda University. The iron balancing act: Vegetarians may have the edge. In *Nutr Health Letter,* www.llu.edu/llu/vegetarian/iron.htm.

Lonsdale D, Shamberger R. Red cell transketolase as an indicator of nutritional deficiency. *Am J Clin Nutr* 1980; 33: 205–11.

Maes M et al. Lower serum vitamin E concentrations in major depression: Another marker of lowered antioxidant defenses in that illness. *J Affect Disorder* 2000 Jun; 58(3): 241–6.

Markowitz JS, DeVane CL. The emerging recognition of herb–drug interactions with a focus on St. John's wort (*Hypericum perforatum*). *Psychopharmacol Bull* 2001 winter; 35(1): 53–64.

McLeod MN, Gaynes BN, Golden RN. Chromium potentiation of antidepressant pharmacotherapy for dysthymic disorder in 5 patients. *J Clin Psychiatry* 1999; 60(4): 237–40.

McLeod MN, Golden RN. Chromium treatment of depression. *Int J Neuropsychopharmacol* 2000 Dec; 3(4): 311–4.

Morris MS et al. Depression and folate status in the US population. *Psychother Psychosom* 2003 Mar–Apr; 72(2): 59–60.

Murray M. *Ginkgo biloba* extract versus phosphatidylserine in treatment of depression and Alzheimer's disease. *Am J Nat Med* 1995 Dec; 2(10): 8–9.

Schubert H, Halama P. Depressive episode primarily unresponsive to therapy in elderly patients: Efficacy of *Ginkgo biloba* extract (EGb 761) in combination with antidepressants. *Geriatr Forsch* 1993; 3: 45–53.

Sher L. Role of thyroid hormones in the effects of selenium on mood, behavior, and cognitive function. *Med Hypotheses* 2001 Jul; 59(1): 480–3.

———. Role of selenium depletion in the effects of dialysis on mood and behavior. *Med Hypotheses* 2002 Jul; 59(1): 89–91.

Shevtsov VA et al. A randomized trial of two different doses of a SHR-5 *Rhodiola rosea* extract vs placebo and control of capacity for mental work. *Phytomedicine* 2003 Mar; 10(2–3): 95–105.

Szegedi A et al. Acute treatment of moderate to severe depression with hypericum extract WS 5570 (St John's wort): Randomised controlled double blind non-inferiority trial versus paroxetine. *BMJ*, www.bmj.com.

Tolmunen T et al. Dietary folate and the risk of depression in Finnish middle-aged men. *Psychother Psychosom* 2004 Nov–Dec; 73(6): 334–9.

Vogel G. Pharmacology: A worrisome side effect of an antianxiety remedy. *Sci* 2001; 291: 37.

Vohra M et al. Folic acid deficiency, www.emedicine.com/med/topic802.htm.

Wright JV. Why you need 83 times more of this essential, cancer-fighting nutrient than the "experts" say you do. *Nutrition and Healing* 2005 May; 12(4): 1–4.

Young SN, Ghadrian AM. Folic acid and psychopathology. *Prog Neuropsychopharmacol Biol Psychiatry* 1989; 13: 841–63.


## CHAPTER 7: Eat Your Way Out of Depression

AHA Scientific Statement. *Circulation* 2002; 106: 2747, http://circ.ahajournals.org/cgi/content/full/106/21/2747#TBL3.

Braly J, Hoggan R. *Dangerous Grains: Why Gluten Cereal Grains May Be Hazardous to Your Health.* New York: Avery, 2002.

Fallon S. *Nourishing Traditions: The Cookbook That Challenges Politically Correct Nutrition and the Diet Dictocrats*, 2nd ed. San Diego: ProMotion Publishing, 1999.

Gottschall E. *Breaking the Vicious Cycle: Intestinal Health Through Diet.* Ontario, Canada: Kirkton Press, 1994, 2004.

Mondoa EI, Kitei M. *Sugars That Heal: The New Healing Science of Glyconutrients.* New York: Ballantine Books, 2002.

Roberts HJ. *Aspartame (Nutrasweet): Is It Safe?* Philadelphia: Charles Press, 1992.

Ross J. *The Diet Cure.* New York: Penguin Putnam, 2000.

Schmid RF. *Traditional Foods Are Your Best Medicine: Improving Health and Longevity with Native Nutrition.* Rochester, VT: Healing Arts Press, 1987, 1994, 1997.

————. *The Untold Story of Milk: Green Pastures, Contented Cows and Raw Dairy Products.* New York: NewTrends Publishing, 2004.

Zubay GL, Parson WW, Vance DE. *Principles of Biochemistry.* Dubuque, IA: Wm. C. Brown, 1995.


## CHAPTER 8: Rid Your Body of Mood-Altering Toxins

American Dental Association Council on Scientific Affairs. 1998 report.

American Gastroenterological Association, www.gastro.org/clinical Res/brochures/ibs.html.

American Heart Association. Study presented at the AHA Asia Pacific Scientific Forum, April 2002, www.sciencedaily.com/releases/2002/04/020429073754.htm.

Bittner AC et al. Behavior effects of low level mercury exposure among dental professionals. *Neurotoxicology Teratology*, 1998; 20(4): 429–39.

Bock K. *The Road to Immunity: How to Survive and Thrive in a Toxic World*. New York: Pocket Books, 1997.

Clark J. Interviewed by Richard Passwater, Lipoic Acid Basics. HealthWorld Online, www.healthy.net/scr/interview.asp?PageType=Interview&ID=160.

Crawford AP. Germ-free nation: Is our obsession with cleanliness beginning to backfire? *Vegetarian Times* 2004 Jul–Aug.

Daunderer M. Improvement of nerve and immunological damages after amalgam removal. *Am J Probiotic Dentistry Medicine* 1991 Jan.

Echeverria D et al. Neurobehavioral effects from exposure to dental amalgam. *FASEBJ* 1998 Aug; 12(11): 971–80.

Eggleston DW, Nylander M. Correlation of dental amalgam with mercury in brain tissue. *J Prosthetic Dent* 1987; 58.

Gay DD, Cox RD, Reinhard JW. Chewing releases mercury from fillings. *Lancet* 1979 May 5.

Harrison IA. Some electrochemical features of the in vivo corrosion of dental amalgams. *J Appl Electrochem* 1989; 19: 301–10.

Hubbard LR. *Purification: An Illustrated Answer to Drugs*. Los Angeles: Bridge Publications, 1990.

———. *Clear Body Clear Mind: The Effective Purification Program*. Los Angeles: Bridge Publications, 2002.

Hultberg B, Andersson A, Isaksson A. Lipoic acid increases glutathione production and enhances the effect of mercury in human cell lines. *Toxicology* 2002 Jun 14; 175(1–3): 103–10.

Jedrychowski W et al. Estimated risk for altered fetal growth resulting from exposure to fine particles during pregnancy. *Environ Health Perspect* 2004 Oct; 112(14): 1398–402.

Kampe T et al. Personality traits of adolescents with intact and repaired dentitions. *Acta Odont Scand* 1986; 44: 95.

Kishi R et al. Residual neurobehavioral effects of chronic exposure to mercury vapor. *Occupat Environ Med* 1994; 1: 35–41.

Liang YX et al. Psychological effects of low exposure to mercury vapor. *Environ Med Res* 1993; 60(2): 320–7.

Lichtenberg HJ. Elimination of symptoms by removal of dental amalgam from mercury poisoned patients. *J Orthomol Med* 1993; 8: 145–8.

———. Symptoms before and after proper amalgam removal in relation to serum-globulin reaction to metals. *J Orthomol Med* 1996; 11(4): 195–203.

Malt UF et al. Physical and mental problems attributed to dental amalgam fillings. *Psychosom Med* 1997; 59: 32–41.

Marek M. Dissolution of mercury vapor in simulated oral environments. *Dent Mater* 1997 Sep; 13(5): 312–5.

Mercola J, Klinghardt D. Mercury toxicity and systemic elimination agents. *J Nutr Environ Med* 2001 March.

O'Carroll RE, Masterson G, Dougall N, et al. The neuropsychiatric sequelae of mercury poisoning: The mad hatter's disease revisited. *Br J Psychiatry* 1995; 67: 95–8.

Park JW, Park MO. Mechanism of metal ion binding to chitosan in solution, cooperative inter- and intramolecular chelations. *Bull Korean Chem Soc* 1984; 5(3): 108.

Perera FP et al. Molecular evidence of an interaction for the prenatal environmental exposure and birth outcomes in multiethnic populations. *Environ Health Perspect* 2004 April; 112 (5): 626–30.

Rapp D. *Is This Your Child's World? How You Can Fix the Schools and Homes That Are Making Your Children Sick.* See www.tcwell ness.com/issues/1998/04/3.html.

Siblerud RL et al. Psychometric evidence that mercury from dental fillings may be a factor in depression, anger, and anxiety. *Psychol Rep* 1994 Feb; 74(1): 67–80.

WebMD, Glutathione: New supplement on the block, www.nutri tionadvisor.com/web_md.htm.

Weiner JA, Nylander M. An estimation of the uptake of mercury from amalgam fillings based on urinary excretion of mercury in Swedish subjects. *Sci Total Environ* 1995 Jun 30; 168(3): 255–65.

## CHAPTER 9: Harness Your Hormones

Akwa Y et al. Neurosteroids: Biosynthesis, metabolism and function of pregnenolone and dehydroepiandrosterone in the brain. *J Steroid Biochem Molec Biol* 1991; 40(1–3): 71–81.

Arendt J. Melatonin—a new probe in psychiatric investigation? *Br J Psychiatry* 1989; 155: 585–90.

Ashman SB. Stress hormone levels of children of depressed mothers. *Dev Psychopathol* 2002; 14(2): 333–49.

Barrett-Connor E et al. Endogenous levels of dehydroepiandros- terone sulfate, but not other sex hormones, are associated with depressed mood in older women: The Rancho Bernardo Study. *J Am Geriatr Soc* 1999 Jun; 47(6): 685–91.

Bloch M et al. Dehydroepiandrosterone treatment for midlife dys- thymia. *Biol Psychiatry* 1999 Jun 15; 45(12): 1533–41.

Brown RP et al. Depressed mood and reality disturbance correlate with decreased nocturnal melatonin in depressed patients. *Acta Psychiatr Scand* 1987; 76(3): 272–5.

Cohen LS et al. Short-term use of estradiol for depression in peri- menopausal and postmenopausal women: A preliminary report. *Am J Psychiatry* 2003; 160(8): 1519–22.

Davis SR, Tran J. Testosterone influences libido and well-being in women. *Trends Endocrinol Metab* 2001; 12(1): 33–7.

Freeman EW et al. Hormones and menopausal status as predictors of depression in women in transition to menopause. *Arch Gen Psychiatry* 2004; 61: 62–70.

George MS et al. CSF neuroactive steroids in affective disorders:

Pregnenolone, progesterone and DBI. *Biol Psychiatry* 1994; 35(10): 775–80.

Goodyear IM et al. Adrenal secretion during major depression in 8- to 16-year-olds. *Psychol Med* 1996 Mar; 26(2): 245–56.

Guechot J et al. Simple laboratory test of neuroendocrine disturbance in depression: 11 P.M. saliva cortisol. *Neuropsychobiology* 1987; 18(1): 1–4.

Hendrick V. Hormones for perimenopausal and postmenopausal depression. *Psychiatric Times* 2004 Jan; 21(1).

Hickie I et al. Clinical and subclinical hypothyroidism in patients with chronic and treatment-resistant depression. *Aust NZ J Psychiatry* 1996; 30(2): 246–52.

Lowe-Ponsford FL. Cortisol, stress and depression, www.defeat depression.org/pdf/cortisolstressdepression.pdf.

Margolese HC. The male menopause and mood: Testosterone decline and depression in the aging male—is there a link? *J Geriatr Psychiatry Neurol* 2000; 13(2): 93–101.

Martin R, Gerstung J. *The Estrogen Alternative.* Rochester, VT: Healing Arts Press, 2004.

McK Jefferies W. *Safe Uses of Cortisol.* Springfield, IL: Charles C Thomas, 1981.

Metzger C et al. Sequential appearance and ultrastructure of amphophilic cell foci, adenomas, and carcinomas in the liver of male and female rats treated with dehydroepiandrosterone. *Toxicol Pathol* 1995 Sep–Oct; 23(5): 591–605.

Nemeroff CB. The neurobiology of depression. *Scientific American* 1998; 278(6): 28–35.

Rabkin JG, Wagner GJ, Rabkin R. Testosterone therapy for human immunodeficiency virus-positive men with and without hypogonadism. *J Clin Psychopharmacol* 1999 Feb; 19(1): 19–27.

Recharge with pregnenolone, *Life Extension Magazine* 2004 Jun, www.lef.org/magazine/mag2004/jun2004_report_preg_01.htm.

Samuels MH, McDaniel PA. Thyrotropin levels during hydrocortisone infusions that mimic fasting-induced cortisol elevations: A clinical research center study. *J Clin Endocrinol Metab* 1997 Nov; 82(11): 3700–4.

Schmidt PJ et al. Estrogen replacement in perimenopause-related depression: A preliminary report. *Am J Obstet Gynecol* 2000; 183(2): 414–20.

Schweiger U et al. Testosterone, gonadotropin, and cortisol secretion in male patients with major depression. *Psychosom Med* 1999 May–Jun; 61(3): 292–6.

Seidman SN, Walsh BT. Testosterone and depression in aging men. *Am J Geriatr Psychiatry* 1999 winter; 7(1): 18–33.

Shafii M et al. Nocturnal serum melatonin profile in major depression in children and adolescents. *Arch Gen Psychiatry* 1996; 53(11): 1009–13.

Shealy N. *Natural Progesterone Cream: Safe and Natural Hormone Replacement.* Los Angeles: Keats Publishing, 1999.

Shively CA et al. Social stress-associated depression in adult female cynomolgus monkeys (*Macaca fascicularis*). *Biol Psychol* 2005 Apr; 69(1): 67–84.

Soares CN et al. Efficacy of estradiol for the treatment of depressive disorders in perimenopausal women: A double-blind, randomized, placebo-controlled trial. *Arch Gen Psychiatry* 2001; 58(6): 529–34.

Stagnaro-Green A. Recognizing, understanding, and treating post-partum thyroiditis. *Endocrinol Metab Clin North Am* 2000; 29(2): 417–30, ix.

Steiner M, Dunn E, Born L. Hormones and mood: From menarche to menopause and beyond. *J Affect Disord* 2003 May; 74(1): 67–83.

Thyroid Society. Can depression be caused by thyroid disease?, http://the-thyroid-society.org/faq/33.html.

Weber B et al. Testosterone, androstenedione and dihydrotestosterone concentrations are elevated in female patients with major depression. *Psychoneuroendocrinology* 2000 Nov; 25(8): 765–71.

Weissman MM. Cross-national epidemiology of major depression and bipolar disorder. *JAMA* 1996 July 24–31; 276(4): 293–99.

Wolkowitz OM et al. Double-blind treatment of major depression with DHEA. *Am J Psychiatry* 1999 Apr; 156(4): 646–9.

Zweifel JE, O'Brien WH. A meta-analysis of the effect of hormone replacement therapy upon depressed mood. *Psychoneuro-endocrinology* 1997; 22(3): 189–212. [Published erratum *Psycho-neuroendocrinology* 22(8): 655.]

## CHAPTER 10: Up with Life

Babyak M et al. Exercise treatment for major depression: Mainte-nance of therapeutic benefit at 10 months. *Psychosom Med* 2000 Sep–Oct; 62(5): 633–8.

Brown RP, Gerbarg PL. Sudarshan Kriya yogic breathing in the treatment of stress, anxiety, and depression: Part I: Neurophysio-logic model. *J Altern Complement Med* 2005 Feb; 11(1): 189–201.

DeRubeis RJ et al. Cognitive therapy versus medications in the treatment of moderate to severe depression. *Arch Gen Psychiatry* 2005; 62: 409–16.

Dunn AL et al. Exercise treatment for depression. *Am J Preventive Med* 2005 Jan; 28(1): 1–8.

Epperson C. *J Clin Psychiatry* 2004 Mar; 65: 521–5.

Field T et al. Massage and relaxation therapies' effects on depressed adolescent mothers. *Adolescence* 1996 winter; 31(124): 903–11.

Golden RN et al. The efficacy of light therapy in the treatment of mood disorders: A review and meta-analysis of the evidence. *Am J Psychiatry* 2005 Apr; 162(4): 656–62.

Grossman P et al. Mindfulness-based stress reduction and health benefits: A meta-analysis. *J Psychosom Res* 2004 Jul; 57(1): 35–43.

Harte JL, Eifert GH, Smith R. The effects of running and media-tion on beta-endorphin, corticotropin-releasing hormone and cortisol in plasma, and on mood. *Biol Psychol (Neth)* 1995 Jun; 40(3): 251–65.

Hollon SD et al. Prevention of relapse following cognitive therapy vs medications in moderate to severe depression. *Arch Gen Psychiatry* 2005; 62: 417–22.

Janakiramaiah N, Gangadhar BN, et al. Antidepressant efficacy of Sudarshan Kriya Yoga (SKY) in melancholia: A randomized comparison with electroconvulsive therapy and imipramine. *J Affect Disord* 2000; 57: 255–9.

Jones NA, Field T. Massage and music therapies attenuate frontal EEG asymmetry in depressed adolescents. *Adolescence* 1999 fall; 34(135): 529–34.

Kabat-Zinn, Jon, PhD. Interviewed by Richard Streitfeld, www.kwanumzen.com/primarypoint/v08n2-1991-summer-jonkabatzinn-mindfulmedicine.html.

Khumar SS, Kaur P, Kaur S. Effectiveness of shavasana on depression among university students. *Indian J Clin Psychol* 1993; 20: 82–7.

Lavie CJ et al. Effects of cardiac rehabilitation and exercise training programs in women with depression. *Am J Cardiol* 1999 May 15; 83(10): 1480–3.

Oren DA et al. An open trial of morning light therapy for treatment of antepartum depression. *Am J Psychiatry* 2002 Apr; 159(4): 666–9.

Woolery A, Myers H, Sternlieb B, Zeltzer L. A yoga intervention for young adults with elevated symptoms of depression. *Altern Ther Health Med* 2004 Mar–Apr; 10(2): 60–3.

## CHAPTER 11: Energy Medicine

Allen JJB, Schnyer RN, Hitt SK. The efficacy of acupuncture in the treatment of major depression in women. *Psychological Science* 1998 Sep.

Eich H et al. Acupuncture in patients with minor depressive

episodes and generalized anxiety. *Fortschr Neurol Psychiatr* 2000 Mar; 68(3): 137–44.

Kleijnen J, Knipschild P, ter Riet G. Clinical trials of homeopathy. *BMJ* 1991; 302: 316–23.

Linde K et al. Are the clinical effects of homeopathy placebo effects? A meta-analysis of placebo-controlled trials. *Lancet* 1997; 250: 834–43.

Manber R et al. Alternative treatments for depression: Empirical support and relevance to women. *J Clin Psychiatry* 2002 Jul; 63(7): 628–40.

———. Acupuncture: A promising treatment for depression during pregnancy. *J Affect Disord* 2004 Nov; 83(1): 89–95.

Shore AG. Long-term effects of energetic healing on symptoms of psychological depression and self-perceived stress. *Altern Therapies* 2004 May–Jun; 10(3).

## CHAPTER 12: Psychotropic Drugs: What's the Story?

Angell M. *The Truth About Drug Companies: How They Deceive Us and What to Do About It.* New York: Random House, 2004.

Angell M, Kassirer JP. Editorial comment. *New England J Med* 1998; 339: 839–41.

Breggin PR. *Talking Back to Prozac.* New York: St. Martin's Paperbacks, 1994.

———. *The Anti-Depressant Fact: What Your Doctor Won't Tell You About Prozac, Zoloft, Paxil, Celexa and Luvox.* Cambridge, MA: Perseus Publishers, 2001.

FDA black box warning on antidepressants creates concerns for clinicians. *Neuropsychiatry Rev* 2004 Dec; 5(9): www.neuro psychiatryreviews.com/dec04/npr_dec04_FDAblackbox.html.

FDA Talk Paper, 2003 Jan 13.

Glenmullen J. *Prozac Backlash: Overcoming the Dangers of Prozac, Zoloft, Paxil, and Other Antidepressants with Safe, Effective Alternatives.* New York: Touchstone, 2000.

Hardy P. The integration of nutraceutical with pharmaceutical ther-
    apy: A functional neuropsychiatric approach to autism. Syllabus
    from DAN! Conference. Quincy, MA, 2005 spring.

*New York Times.* Odds are the drug industry is paying off your doc-
    tor. 2004 Feb 25, www.nytimes.com/2004/02/24/health/
    policy/24ESSA.html.

*Psychiatric News* 2004 Aug 6; 39(15): 39, http://pn.psychiatry
    online.org/cgi/content/full/39/15/39-b.

Red Flags. 2002 Aug 15, www.redflagsweekly.com/Thursday_
    report/2002_august15.html.

# Appendix:
# Organizations and Resources

―――――――― ⚜ ――――――――

## Practitioner Referrals

The following organizations list practitioners who have an interest in orthomolecular, complementary, alternative, integrative, holistic, naturopathic, functional, or environmental medicine. Each organization has its own criteria for listing, and each one presents varying degrees of information about the practitioners' background and training. The background, training, and scope of practice vary considerably from practitioner to practitioner. Selecting a practitioner from the database of any one of these organizations does not replace a thorough investigation of your chosen clinician's professional degree and training, clinical experience, scope of practice, participation (or not) in the reimbursement system, malpractice coverage, and similar criteria. The author and publisher therefore take no responsibility for any problems that arise in your choosing a practitioner. This information is presented for informational purposes only; it is the responsibility of the patient to do a full investigation before choosing a practitioner.

**American Academy of Environmental Medicine**
East Kellogg Ste 625
Wichita KS 67207
316-684-5500
www.aaem.com

**American College for Advancement in Medicine**
  23121 Verdugo Dr Ste 204
  Laguna Hills CA 92653
  800-532-3688
  www.acam.org

**Institute for Functional Medicine**
  4411 Pt Fosdick Dr NW Ste 305
  PO Box 1697
  Gig Harbor WA 98335
  800-228-0622
  www.functionalmedicine.org

# General Information

Note: Some of these websites also have a database of practitioner referrals.

**Alternative Medicine Resources**
  www.alternativemedicine.com

**Doctor's Medical Library**
  www.medical-library.net/specialties/framer.html?/specialtiesd/
  orthomolecular_medicine.html

**Health Research Institute and Pfeiffer Treatment Center**
  4575 Weaver Pkwy
  Warrenville IL 60555-4039
  630-505-0300
  www.hriptc.org

**Linus Pauling Institute**
  Oregon State University
  571 Weniger Hall
  Corvallis, OR 97331-6512
  541-737-5075
  http://lpi.oregonstate.edu/

**Orthomolecular Medicine Online**
www.orthomed.org

**Orthomolecular.Org**
3100 N Hillside Ave
Wichita KS 67219
316-682-3100
http://orthomolecular.org

**Worldwide Health Center**
www.worldwidehealthcenter.net/directory-44.html
An alternative and complementary medicine directory.

## Acupuncture

**American Academy of Medical Acupuncture**
4929 Wilshire Blvd Ste 428
Los Angeles CA 90010
323-937-5514
www.medicalacupuncture.org

**National Certification Commission for Acupuncture and Oriental Medicine**
11 Canal Center Plz Ste 300
Alexandria VA 22314
703-548-9004
www.nccaom.org

## Amalgam Removal

**International Academy of Oral Medicine and Toxicology**
www.iaomt.org

**American Academy of Biological Dentistry**
www.biologicaldentistry.org

## Colon Hydrotherapy

Each of the following sites offers a directory of professional colon hydrotherapists:

http://colonhydrotherapyonline.com/directory

**Colon Therapist Network**
http://colonhealth.net/therapist/sample.html

www.byregion.net/healers/categorypages/Colonic+Hydrotherapy
.html

## Diet Information

**Celiac Sprue Association**
877-CSA-4CSA
www.csaceliacs.org
Offers information and a 370-plus-page resource called *CSA Gluten-Free Product Listing.*

**The Specific Carbohydrate Diet**
www.scdiet.org

**Gluten-Free Pantry**
PO Box 840
Gastonbury CT 06033
Customer service: 860-633-3826
www.glutenfree.com

**Gluten-Free Diet Support Center**
www.celiac.com
Resource for gluten-free and casein-free information and foods.

**Gluten-Free Mall**
PO Box 279
Gardena CA 90248
www.glutenfreemall.com
All online ordering; no phone orders.

# Fluoride

**Fluoride Action Network**
802-355-0999
www.fluoridealert.org

www.holisticmed.com/fluoride
An extensive list of resources.

**Citizens for Safe Drinking Water**
www.keepers-of-the-well.org/Introduction.html

www.garynull.com/documents/Dental/Fluoride/fluoride_index.htm

# Homeopathy

www.homeopathy-cures.com/html/referrals_to_homeopaths.html
Referrals to classical homeopaths.

**National Center for Homeopathy**
877-624-0613
www.homeopathic.org
An organization for homeopaths, but it answers questions from
the public.

**American Institute of Homeopaths**
www.homeopathyusa.org
A professional association of medical homeopaths, it publishes a
directory of medical homeopaths.

**Homeopathic Academy of Naturopathic Physicians**
www.hanp.net
Provides a list of naturopathic physicians who practice
homeopathy.

**North American Society of Homeopaths**
www.homeopathy.org
Provides a list of certified homeopaths.

# Iodine Research

**The Iodine Project**
www.optimox.com; click on Iodine Research
The full text of all of Dr. Guy Abraham's papers.

# Laboratories That Specialize in One or More Orthomolecular Procedures

**Doctor's Data, Inc.**
PO Box 111
West Chicago IL 60186
United States and Canada 800-323-2784
www.doctorsdata.com/Contact.htm

**Great Smokies Diagnostic Laboratory/Genovations**
63 Zillicoa St
Asheville NC 28801
800-522-4762
https://www.gsdl.com/home/

**Metametrix**
4855 Peachtree Industrial Blvd Ste 201
Norcross GA 30092
800-221-4640 or 770-446-5483
www.metametrix.com

**NeuroScience Inc.**
www.neuroscienceinc.com
Information on neurotransmitter testing, amino acid therapy, hormone therapy.

# Light Therapy

**Light Therapy Products**
612 S Ives Ln N
Plymouth MN 55442
800-486-6723
www.lighttherapyproducts.com

**Alaska Northern Lights**
PO Box 1801
Homer AK 99603
800-880-6953
www.alaskanorthernlights.com

**Enviro-Med**
1600 SE 141st Ave
Vancouver WA 98683
800-222-DAWN
www.bio-light.com

## Massage

**American Massage Therapy Foundation**
500 Davis St Ste 900
Evanston IL 60201
847-869-5019
www.massagetherapyfoundation.org

## Naturopathic Physicians (Including Referrals)

**The American Association of Naturopathic Physicians (AANP)**
www.naturopathic.org

## Nutrients/Nutraceuticals

**Allergy Research Group**
2300 N Loop Rd
Alameda CA 94502
800-545-9960; worldwide 1-510-263-2000
www.allergyresearchgroup.com

**Garden of Life**
5500 Village Blvd Ste 202

West Palm Beach FL 33407
561-748-2477
www.gardenoflifeusa.com
Whole food supplements, probiotics.

## Good Earth Natural Foods Company
6350 Guilford Ave
Indianapolis IN 46220
317-254-8604
www.good-earth.com
Whole food supplements.

## Juice Plus
www.juiceplus.com
Information about concentrated fruit and vegetable
supplements.

## GlycoScience: The Nutrition Science Site
www.glycoscience.org
Information on essential sugars.

## Mannatech
600 S Royal Ln Ste 200
Coppell TX 75019
972-471-8111
www.mannatech.com
Essential sugar supplements.

## NeuroScience Inc.
www.neuroscienceinc.com
Information on neurotransmitter testing, amino acid therapy,
hormone therapy, and exclusive nutraceuticals.

## Xymogen Inc.
725 S Kirkman Rd
Orlando FL 32811
800-647-6100
Exclusive professional formulas.

# Reiki

**International Association of Reiki Professionals**
PO Box 104
Harrisville NH 03450
603-881-8838
www.iarp.org
A directory of Reiki professionals in the United States and the world.

**The Reiki Alliance**
204 N Chestnut St
Kellogg ID 83837
208-783-3535
www.reikialliance.com
A directory of Reiki professionals in the United States.

# Support Groups/Chats

**Depression and Bipolar Support Alliance**
www.dbsalliance.org
Offers online support groups and a directory of local support groups.

**Healthy Place**
www.healthyplace.com/communities/depression/site/comm
_calender.htm
Offers online chats and group support meetings.

# Visualization/Guided Imagery

**Guided Imagery Inc.**
2937 Lamplight Ln
Willoughby Hills OH 44094
440-944-9292
www.guidedimageryinc.com
CDs and tapes.

**Peter S. Reznik, PhD**
  *Staying Healthy in a Stressful World: A Comprehensive Manual for
  Self Mastery and Freedom from Stress* CD
  212-838-6809
  www.drpeterreznik.com

## Water Filters

**Crystal Quest**
  Abode Water Filters
  Hawley MA 01339
  413-339-5346
  www.purewaterabode.com/CrystalQuest.htm

**DoultonUSA**
  19541 Cherry Hill Rd
  Southfield MI 48076
  888-664-3336
  www.doultonusa.com

**Pure Water Systems**
  5707 238th Pl NE
  Redmond WA 98053
  866-444-9926
  www.purewatersystems.com

**Wholly Water filtration system**
  Life Streams International Manufacturing Co.
  Westmoreland NY 13490
  800-76-WATER
  www.wholly-water.com/fluoride.htm

# Glossary

**Acetylcholine.** A neurotransmitter that is involved in many functions, including mood, sleep, cognition, and the functioning of several organs, including the heart and liver.

**Adaptogen.** A substance that helps bring a process or function back toward normal.

**Adrenal cortex.** The outer portion of the adrenal glands; it produces steroid hormones that regulate fat and carbohydrate metabolism as well as water and salt balance.

**Adrenal fatigue.** A syndrome in which the adrenal glands have a reduced ability to respond adequately to stress.

**Adrenal glands.** A pair of glands, one atop each of the kidneys, that produce hormones that control heart rate, blood pressure, mineral levels, and other vital functions.

**Adrenaline.** See *epinephrine.*

**Adrenal medulla.** The inner part of the adrenal gland that produces epinephrine (adrenaline) and norepinephrine (noradrenaline).

**Adrenocorticotropic hormone (ACTH).** A hormone secreted by the pituitary to stimulate the production of cortisol and other adrenal hormones.

**Amylase.** An enzyme that digests carbohydrates.

**Bile.** A liquid produced in the liver, stored in the gallbladder, and secreted into the small intestine that helps to emulsify and therefore digest fats.

**Bioavailable.** Is readily utilized by the body.

**Bipolar disorder.** A mental disorder characterized by rapid mood swings.

**Blood–brain barrier.** A specialized network of blood vessels and cells that filters blood flowing to the brain and prevents the passage of certain substances into the brain.

**Candidiasis.** Overgrowth of the *Candida albicans* yeast in the gastrointestinal tract or other areas of the body. Candidiasis tends to occur when the normal balance of bacteria in the gut is compromised.

**Chelation therapy.** A form of therapy in which a substance that binds with heavy metals is introduced into the body to help eliminate the metals in the urine.

**Corticotropin-releasing factor (CRF).** The hormone secreted by the hypothalamus that stimulates the pituitary to produce adrenocorticotropic hormone.

**Cortisol.** A hormone produced by the adrenal cortex; often referred to as the stress hormone.

**Cyclothymia.** A milder form of bipolar disorder, it is characterized by less dramatic mood swings and less severe symptoms.

**Dehydroepiandrosterone (DHEA).** A hormone secreted by the adrenal glands that serves as a precursor to sex hormones and other hormones in the body.

**Detoxification.** A process that removes toxins from the body.

**Dysthymia.** A mood disorder characterized by long periods of chronic depression alternating with brief periods of normal mood.

**Endorphins.** Any of a group of peptide hormones that bind to opiate receptors and are found mainly in the brain. Endorphins reduce the sensation of pain and affect emotions.

**Enkephalins.** Either of two closely related pentapeptides (five amino acids chained together) having opiate qualities and occurring especially in the brain and spinal cord.

**Epinephrine.** A hormone produced by the medulla of the adrenal gland. Increased secretion of epinephrine (also known as adrenaline) occurs during stressful situations and can result in a quickened heart rate, increased respiration, and other effects.

**Essential fatty acids (EFAs).** Unsaturated fatty acids that are essential to human health but cannot be manufactured by the body. The three types of EFAs are arachidonic acid, linoleic acid, and linolenic acid.

**Hyperthyroidism.** A condition in which production of thyroid hormones is above normal. Symptoms may include rapid heartbeat, sweating, weight loss, insomnia, and protruding eyeballs.

**Hypothalamus.** A gland located in the brain below the thalamus and above the pituitary gland. It regulates thirst, hunger, and body temperature, among other functions.

**Hypothyroidism.** A condition in which production of thyroid hormones is below normal. Symptoms may include depression, intolerance of cold, fatigue, constipation, and thinning and/or brittle nails and hair.

**Lipase.** An enzyme that digests fats.

**Manic depressive illness.** A disease or condition during which a person has extended periods of mood swings from mania to depression.

**Monoamine.** An amine compound containing one amino group, especially a compound that functions as a neurotransmitter. A class of neurotransmitters and hormones that includes catecholamines (dopamine, epinephrine, norepinephine) and the indoleamines (serotonin, melatonin).

**Monoamine oxidase.** An enzyme in the cells of most tissues that catalyzes the oxidative deamination of monoamines such as serotonin and other monoamine neurotransmitters.

**Monoamine oxidase inhibitors.** Any of a class of antidepressant and hypotensive drugs that block the action of monoamine oxidase in the brain, thereby allowing the accumulation of monoamines such as norepinephrine and serotonin.

**Neuron.** An impulse-conducting brain cell. There are many types of neurons in the brain.

**Neurotransmitter.** Any one of many chemicals that transmit signals between neurons. Examples of neurotransmitters include serotonin, dopamine, epinephrine, and norepinephrine.

**Noradrenaline.** See *norepinephrine.*

**Norepinephrine.** A neurotransmitter secreted by sympathetic nervous system neurons.

**Opioid.** A drug, hormone, or other chemical substance that has sedative or narcotic effects similar to those of opium (heroin) or its derivatives. Painkilling action.

**Opioid receptor.** Receptors on cells, especially in the brain, that are stimulated by opioids.

**Peptide.** Any of various natural or synthetic compounds containing two or more amino acids linked by the carboxyl group of one amino acid and the amino group of another.

**Probiotic.** A microbe that helps prevent disease. The best-known probiotic is *Lactobacillus acidophilus*, which helps maintain healthful bacteria in the intestinal tract.

**Protease.** An enzyme that helps digest protein and breaks it into peptides.

**Psychotropic drug.** Any drug that is capable of affecting the mind, behavior, and emotions.

**Receptors.** Special chemical structures located on the surface of neurons; they receive signals from other neurons. A receptor must be activated for the signals to get through.

**Selective serotonin reuptake inhibitor (SSRI).** A class of drugs, such as fluoxetine (Prozac), that inhibit the reuptake of serotonin by the neuron that secretes it, resulting in an increase of the neurotransmitter in the synapse. They are often used in the treatment of depression.

**Synapse.** The space, or gap, between neurons. This is the space across which neurotransmitters travel to the adjoining neuron to stimulate it.

**Thyroxin.** The major hormone secreted by the thyroid gland.

# Suggested Reading

꧁

## Alternative/Complementary Treatments

Bauer, Matthew. *The Healing Power of Acupressure and Acupuncture.* New York: Avery, 2005.

Baumel, Syd. *Dealing with Depression Naturally.* New York: McGraw-Hill, 1995.

Eden, Donna, and David Feinstein. *Energy Medicine: Balancing Your Body's Energies for Optimum Health, Joy and Vitality.* New York: Penguin, 2000.

Epstein, Gerald. *Healing Visualizations: Creating Health Through Imagery.* New York: Bantam, 1989.

Gawain, Shakti. *Creative Visualization: Use the Power of Your Imagination to Create What You Want in Your Life,* 25th anniversary edition. New York: New World Library, 2002.

Gerber, Richard. *Vibrational Medicine: The #1 Handbook of Subtle Energy Therapies.* Rochester, VT: Inner Traditions International, 2001.

Hendrix, Harville. *Getting the Love You Want: A Guide for Couples.* New York: Henry Holt and Company, 1988; first Owl Books edition, 2001.

Hobday, Richard. *The Healing Sun: Sunlight and Health in the 21st Century.* New York: Findhorn, 2000.

Holick, M. *The UV Advantage.* New York: I Books, Simon & Schuster, 2004.

Jahnke, Roger. *The Healer Within: Using Traditional Chinese Tech-*

*niques to Release Your Body's Own Medicine.* New York: Harper-Collins, 1998.

Kabat-Zinn, Jon. *Mindfulness Meditation.* Niles, IL: Nightingale Conant, 2002.

Kidson, Ruth. *Acupuncture for Everyone: What It Is, How It Works, and How It Can Help You.* Rochester, VT: Inner Traditions International, 2001.

Liberman, Jacob. *Light: Medicine of the Future.* Rochester, VT: Bear & Company, 1990.

Lockie, Andrew, and Nicola Geddes. *Natural Health Complete Guide to Homeopathy,* 2nd ed. New York: DK Publishing, 2000.

McCabe, Ed. *Flood Your Body with Oxygen.* Morrisville, NY: Energy Publications, 2003.

Murray, Steve. *Reiki: The Ultimate Guide.* Body & Mind Productions, 2004; www.healingreiki.com.

Oschman, James L. *Energy Medicine: The Scientific Basis.* New York: Elsevier, 2000.

Ott, John. *Health and Light: The Effects of Natural and Artificial Light on Man and Other Living Things.* Columbus, OH: Ariel Press, 2000.

Robbins, Jim. *Symphony in the Brain: The Evolution of the New Brain Wave Biofeedback.* New York: Grove/Atlantic, 2001.

Saul, Andrew. *Doctor Yourself: Natural Healing That Works.* North Bergen, NJ: Basic Health Publications, 2003.

Ullman, Dana. *The Consumer's Guide to Homeopathy.* New York: Penguin, 1995.

Weintraub, Amy. *Yoga for Depression: A Compassionate Guide to Relieving Suffering Through Yoga.* New York: Broadway Books, 2003.

Weiss, Brian L. *Meditation.* Carlsbad, CA: Hay House Inc., 2002.

## Depression: Overview/General Treatment Approaches

Amen, Daniel G. *Change Your Brain, Change Your Life: The Breakthrough Program for Conquering Anxiety, Depression, Obsession, Anger, and Impulsiveness.* New York: Three Rivers Press, 1999.

Cousens, Gabriel. *Depression-Free for Life.* New York: HarperCollins, 2000.

Ross, Julia. *The Mood Cure.* New York: Penguin Putnam, 2002.

Wright, Jesse H., and Monica Ramirez Basco. *Getting Your Life Back: The Complete Guide to Recovery from Depression.* New York: Simon & Schuster, 2001.

## Hormones

Berkson, D. Lindsey. *Hormone Deception: How Everyday Foods and Products Are Disrupting Your Hormones—and How to Protect Yourself and Your Family.* Chicago: Contemporary Books, 2000.

Martin, Raquel, and Judi Gerstung. *The Estrogen Alternative: A Guide to Natural Hormonal Balance*, 4th ed. Rochester, VT: Healing Arts Press, 2005.

McK. Jefferies, W. *Safe Uses of Cortisol.* Springfield, IL: Charles C Thomas, 1981.

Reiter, Russel J., and Jo Robinson. *Your Body's Natural Wonder Drug: Melatonin.* New York: Bantam Books, 1995.

Shames, Richard L., and Karilee Hao Shames. *Thyroid Power: 10 Steps to Total Health.* New York: HarperCollins, 2002.

## Medications

Breggin, Peter R. *The Anti-Depressant Fact: What Your Doctor Won't Tell You About Prozac, Zoloft, Paxil, Celexa and Luvox.* Cambridge, MA: Perseus Publishers, 2001.

———. *Talking Back to Prozac.* New York: St. Martin's, 1994.

Cohen, Jay S. *Overdose: The Case Against Drug Companies.* New York: Jerome P. Tarcher/Putnam, 2001.

Dreyfus, Jack. *A Remarkable Medicine Has Been Overlooked.* New York: Lantern Books, 2000.

———. *The Story of a Remarkable Medicine.* New York: Lantern Books, 2003.

Glenmullen, Joseph. *Prozac Backlash: Overcoming the Dangers of Prozac, Zoloft, Paxil, and Other Antidepressants with Safe, Effective Alternatives.* New York: Touchstone, 2000.


## Nutrition and Supplement Issues

Braly, James, and Ron Hoggan. *Dangerous Grains: Why Gluten Cereal Grains May Be Hazardous to Your Health.* New York: Avery, 2002.

Braverman, Eric R., and Ken Blum. *The Healing Nutrients Within.* North Bergen, NJ: Basic Health Publications, 2002.

Brown, Richard, Carol Colman, and Teodoro Bottiglieri. *Stop Depression Now: SAM-e, the Breakthrough Supplement That Works as Well as Prescription Drugs in Half the Time . . . With No Side Effects.* New York: Penguin, 1999.

Brown, Richard P., and Patricia L. Gerbarg. *Rhodiola Revolution.* Emmaus, PA: Rodale, Inc., 2004.

Brownstein, David. *Iodine: Why You Need It, Why You Can't Live Without It.* West Bloomfield, MI: Medical Alternative Press, 2004.

Casper, David, and Thomas Stone. *Modern Foods: The Sabotage of Earth's Food Supply.* Scottsdale, AZ: Centerpoint Press, 2002.

Chaitow, Leon. *Thorson's Guide to Amino Acids.* London: HarperCollins, 1991.

Challen, Jack, ed. *User's Guide to Nutritional Supplements.* Ontario, Canada: Fitzhenry & Whiteside, 2004.

Dubouch, George. *Science or Miracle? The Metabolic Glyconutritional Discovery.* Talent, OR: Innerlife Foundation, 2003.

Elkins, Rita M. H. *Miracle Sugars.* Orem, UT: Woodland Publishing, 2003.

Fallon, Sally. *Nourishing Traditions: The Cookbook That Challenges Politically Correct Nutrition and the Diet Dictocrats,* 2nd ed. San Diego: ProMotion Publishing, 1999.

Gottschall, Elaine. *Breaking the Vicious Cycle: Intestinal Health Through Diet.* Ontario, Canada: Kirkton Press, Ltd., 1994, 2004.

Grazi, Sol, and Marie Costa. *SAMe: The Safe and Natural Way to Combat Depression and Relieve the Pain of Osteoarthritis.* Rocklin, CA: Prima Health Publishing, 1999.

Haas, Elson M. *Staying Healthy with Nutrition.* Berkeley, CA: Ten Speed Press, 1990.

Lesser, Michael, with Colleen Kapklein. *The Brain Chemistry Diet.* New York: Putnam, 2002.

Mondoa, Emil I., and Mindy Kitei. *Sugars That Heal: The New Healing Science of Glyconutrients.* New York: Ballantine Books, 2002.

Napier, Kristine. *The Omega-3 Advantage.* New York: Barnes & Noble, 2003.

Price, Weston A. *Nutrition and Physical Degeneration.* New Canaan, CT: Keats Publishing, Inc., 1945, 1970, 1989.

Ross, Julia. *The Diet Cure.* New York: Penguin Putnam, 2000.

Schmid, Ronald F. *Traditional Foods Are Your Best Medicine: Improving Health and Longevity with Native Nutrition.* Rochester, VT: Healing Arts Press, 1987, 1994, 1997.

Stoll, Andrew L. *The Omega-3 Connection.* New York: Simon & Schuster, 2001.

## Other Medical Conditions

Edelson, Stephen B., and Deborah Mitchell. *What Your Doctor May Not Tell You About Autoimmune Disorders.* New York: Warner, 2003.

Goldberg, Burton, and Larry Triviera Jr. *Chronic Fatigue, Fibromyalgia & Lyme Disease.* Berkeley, CA: Celestial Arts, 2004.

Kirby, David. *Evidence of Harm: Mercury in Vaccines and the Autism Epidemic: A Medical Controversy.* New York: St. Martin's Press, 2005.

Lee, John, MD. *What Your Doctor May* Not *Tell You About Breast Cancer.* New York: Warner, 2002.

Shomon, Mary J. *Living Well with Graves' Disease and Hyperthyroidism.* New York: HarperCollins, 2005.

Wilson, James. *Adrenal Fatigue: The 21st Century Stress Syndrome.* Petaluma, CA: Smart Publications, 2001.

## Toxins and Detoxification

Blaylock, Russel L. *Excitotoxins: The Taste That Kills.* Santa Fe, NM: Health Press, 1997.

Bower, Lynn Marie. *Creating a Healthy Household.* Bloomington, IN: Healthy House Institute, 2000.

Breiner, Mark A. *Whole Body Dentistry.* Fairfield, CT: Quantum Health Press, 1999.

Bryson, Christopher. *The Fluoride Deception.* New York: Seven Stories Press, 2004.

Cave, Stephanie, MD, and Deborah Mitchell. *What Your Doctor May* Not *Tell You About Children's Vaccinations.* New York: Warner, 2002.

Hubbard, L. Ron. *Purification: An Illustrated Answer to Drugs.* Los Angeles: Bridge Publications, 1990.

————. *Clear Body Clear Mind: The Effective Purification Program.* Los Angeles: Bridge Publications, 2002.

McVicker, Marilyn G. *Sauna Detoxification Therapy: A Guide for the Chemically Sensitive.* Jefferson, NC: McFarland & Co., 1997.

Rapp, Doris. *Our Toxic World: A Wakeup Call.* Buffalo, NY: Environmental Medical Research, 2004.

Roberts, H. J. *Aspartame (Nutrasweet): Is It Safe?* Philadelphia: Charles Press, 1992.

Rogers, Sherry. *Detoxify or Die.* Syracuse, NY: Prestige Publishers, 2002.

# Index

# About the Author

❧

MICHAEL B. SCHACHTER, MD, is a magna cum laude graduate of Columbia College, and received his medical degree from Columbia's Physicians & Surgeons in 1965. He is board certified in psychiatry and has achieved advanced proficiency in chelation therapy from the American College for Advancement in Medicine (ACAM). Dr. Schachter has been involved with alternative and complementary medicine since 1974. He is a recognized leader in orthomolecular psychiatry, nutritional medicine, chelation therapy for cardiovascular disease, and alternative cancer therapies. Coauthor of *Food, Mind and Mood* (1989, 1987) and author of *The Natural Way to a Healthy Prostate* (Keats, 1995), Dr. Schachter was a major contributor to *Alternative Medicine's Definitive Guide to Cancer* (Future Medicine, 1997). He was president of the American College for Advancement in Medicine from 1989–91 and is the past president of the Foundation for the Advancement of Innovative Medicine (FAIM). A frequent lecturer to both professionals and the public, Dr. Schachter is often a guest on radio and television, speaking about health and related topics.